NOV 2011

POWER
OF DISCARD
VITAMIN D

COLLECTION MANAGEMENT

POWER OF VITAMIN D

NEW SCIENTIFIC RESEARCH LINKS VITAMIN D DEFICIENCY TO
CANCER
HEART DISEASE
DIABETES
HIGH BLOOD PRESSURE
KIDNEY DISEASE
FIBROMYALGIA
CHRONIC FATIGUE
OSTEOPOROSIS
ARTHRITIS
LUPUS
M.S.
ASTHMA
THYROID DISEASES
DENTAL PROBLEMS
PROBLEMS DURING PREGNANCY
PROBLEMS IN NEWBORNS
AND
DEPRESSION.

Learn How You Can Reap Miraculous Health
Benefits Of Vitamin D!

Sarfraz Zaidi, MD

Outskirts Press, Inc.
Denver, Colorado

Disclaimer

The information in this book is true and complete to the best of our knowledge. This book is intended only as an informative guide for those wishing to know more about health issues. The information in this book is not intended to replace the advice of a health care provider. The author and publisher disclaim any liability for the decisions you make based on the information contained in this book. The information provided herein should not be used during any medical emergency or for the diagnosis and treatment of any medical condition. In no way is this book intended to replace, countermand, or conflict with the advice given to by your own health care provider. The information contained in this book is general and is offered with no guarantees on the part of the author or publisher. The author and publisher disclaim all liability in connection with the use of this book. The names and identifying details of people associated with events described in this book have been changed. Any similarity to actual persons is coincidental. Any duplication or distribution of information contained herein is strictly prohibited.

I dedicate this book to my patients,
who have been my great teachers.

Table of Contents

Introduction

For years, Evelyn suffered from body aches and pains as well as lack of energy. She consulted several physicians. One specialist gave her the diagnosis of Fibromyalgia. Another physician told her she had Chronic Fatigue Syndrome. Someone else told her, "It's all in your head." She was told to just live with it.

This advice didn't satisfy Evelyn. "There has to be a better answer," she said to one of her coworkers, who happened to be my patient and had been on the same dreadful road herself until she consulted me. She told Evelyn that her body aches, pains and chronic fatigue had vanished after she finally got the right diagnosis and treatment. Evelyn immediately made an appointment to see me.

"You're my last hope, Doc," Evelyn said during her visit. I could sense utter frustration in her voice. I tested her vitamin D level which turned out to be very low. With proper treatment of vitamin D deficiency, Evelyn was relieved of her symptoms in just three months.

I see patients like Evelyn every day in my practice. What amazes me is that physicians run numerous expensive and complicated tests, but don't think to order the one simple test that could clinch the diagnosis. Sad!

Here's the plain truth. Most physicians don't have adequate knowledge about vitamin D deficiency and its serious consequences. What little they do know about vitamin D deficiency is based on outdated and inaccurate information.

My own journey to "enlightenment about vitamin D" started about ten years ago. I vividly remember the day at a medical conference in the Boston area when an old professor gave an amazing talk about vitamin D deficiency. Not only are humans affected, he brilliantly explained, but even animals can develop vitamin D deficiency and its awful complications. For example, in nature, iguanas spend most of the day sun bathing. In captivity however, they can develop severe deficiency of vitamin D and consequently, their back bones melt away.

This lecture definitely left a mark on me. Like most other doctors, I was taught that vitamin D deficiency occurs primarily in older folks, people living in cold, northern areas and patients on kidney dialysis. However, the professor made it very clear that it is quite prevalent in young active people, as well.

On my flight home, I kept thinking about it. I wondered, "What about people living in warm, sunny places like my hometown in southern California? Are they low in vitamin D?" I was taught that people living in sunny places like California and Florida don't develop vitamin D deficiency. Like a true scientist, I wanted to figure it out myself.

I decided to start checking vitamin D levels in my patients. Was I in for a big surprise! Almost 90% of my patients were low in vitamin D. Most of my patients are active people. They are often involved in all sorts of outdoor activities over the weekends. They are proactive in taking care of their health. They take multivitamins, calcium and vitamin D. They are not elderly shut-ins or kidney dialysis patients. And they live in weather charmed, sunny Southern California.

I started to give my vitamin D deficient patients a dose of vitamin D higher than the recommended dose, while closely monitoring them for vitamin D toxicity. I checked their vitamin D level periodically and adjusted the dose of vitamin D accordingly. I was surprised to find that most people required about <u>five to ten times the recommended dose</u> to achieve a good level of vitamin D.

With proper replacement of vitamin D, I started seeing some amazing results in my patients. Body aches and pains simply disappeared. People who were tired all the time and didn't want to do much made a U-turn. Now they had plenty of energy to participate in their favorite activities. Women with osteoporosis did very well. Their bone density got better and fractures were rare. Diabetics achieved excellent control of their blood sugars. Diabetics are at particularly high risk for heart disease, stroke and cancer, but in my patients, these medical catastrophes were rare occurrences. Patients with thyroid disease felt much better.

I'm not attributing all these great results simply to vitamin D replacement because I have developed my own effective strategies in treating diabetes and thyroid diseases. However, proper vitamin D replacement has been a significant factor in achieving these great results.

In the last few years, many researchers have done excellent work in the field of vitamin D and their findings are in line with my own clinical experience. The relationship of vitamin D deficiency to bone pains, osteoporosis, immune disorders, heart disease, high blood pressure, depression and cancer is well established now. There is also strong evidence to support that vitamin D deficiency may play a significant role in the development of diabetes.

Over the last ten years, my patients have benefited from my strategy of diagnosing and treating vitamin D deficiency. It's time to spread this important knowledge. That's why I decided to write this book.

CHAPTER 1

Why is Vitamin D important?

In the last 20 years, there has been tremendous research in the field of vitamin D. The findings are astounding! We now know that vitamin D affects almost every organ system in the body.

We now know that:

1. Vitamin D plays a vital role in the health of *muscles and bones*. It not only helps in the absorption of calcium and phosphorus from the intestines, but it also exerts a direct effect on the health of the bones. Therefore, vitamin D may prevent as well as treat muscle aches, bone pains, chronic fatigue and osteoporosis.

2. Vitamin D plays a vital role in the normal functioning of the *immune system*. Therefore, vitamin D may prevent as well as treat immune disorders such as asthma, rheumatoid arthritis, Type 1 diabetes, Crohn's disease and Multiple Sclerosis (MS).

3. Vitamin D controls the growth of normal as well as *cancerous cells*. Hence, vitamin D may play an important role in the prevention as well as treatment of various cancers especially cancer of the colon, prostate, pancreas and breast.

4. Vitamin D stimulates the production of *insulin* from insulin - producing cells in the pancreas. It also reduces *insulin resistance*. Therefore, vitamin D may help in the prevention

as well as treatment of Type 2 diabetes.

5. Vitamin D inhibits the Renin Angiotensin Aldosterone System (RAAS). Renin is a chemical normally produced in the body. It leads to the production of another chemical, called Angiotensin which is responsible for maintaining your blood pressure. Angiotensin also causes release of another chemical, called Aldosterone which is also involved in maintaining your blood pressure. Together, this system of inter-related chemicals is called Renin Angiotensin Aldosterone System (RAAS). If RAAS becomes overactive, it causes high blood pressure (hypertension), kidney disease and heart failure. Now consider this: *Vitamin D inhibits RAAS*, and therefore, it may prevent *hypertension, kidney disease and heart failure*.

6. Vitamin D may prevent *coronary heart disease* through a number of mechanisms which include inhibition of RAAS, reduction in insulin resistance and prevention of cholesterol deposition in the blood vessel wall.

7. Vitamin D affects the normal function of the skin and therefore can be helpful in the treatment of skin disorders such as *Psoriasis*.

8. Vitamin D affects the health of the teeth and therefore may play an important role in preventing many dental problems.

9. Vitamin D affects one's mood and therefore may play an important role in the prevention and treatment of mood disorders such as *depression*.

Isn't it obvious that vitamin D plays a crucial role in maintaining our health? It's a breakthrough discovery! Now we may truly prevent and treat a number of diseases through proper vitamin D supplementation.

"Why hasn't my Doctor told me about all the beneficial effects of Vitamin D?" ━━━━━━━━━━━━━━━

Unfortunately, this exciting new knowledge about vitamin D hasn't reached the radar screen of most physicians, nor has it reached the curriculum of medical schools. Why? Because no drug company is behind it. It's not a drug. It's cheap and you can obtain it over the counter. Unfortunately, most of our medical research, medical guidelines for practicing physicians and medical knowledge in text books is dependent upon drug companies in one way or another. Sad but true!

It may take years before this revolutionary knowledge finds its way into medical books and physician's offices. But you don't have to wait that long. Get involved in taking charge of your health. Reading this book is a step in the right direction.

In the following chapters, you'll find detailed information on:

A. The remarkable benefits of vitamin D

B. The symptoms and diseases you may have if you are low in vitamin D

C. How to accurately diagnose vitamin D deficiency

D. How to properly treat vitamin D deficiency without worrying about toxicity.

CHAPTER 2

What is Vitamin D?

Most people, including doctors, don't really understand what vitamin D truly is. Why do we have such a limited understanding about vitamin D? In order to answer this question, we need to trace the historic background of our understanding of vitamin D.

The Long Journey to Understanding Vitamin D ━━━━━━

Let me take you back to post-Industrial Revolution Europe, when physicians began to notice a new disease among children living in big industrial cities such as London and Warsaw. These children had stunted growth, muscle wasting and deformed legs. Physicians named this new disease **rickets**, but no one understood the cause of this crippling disease.

Now we look back and realize that these children had little exposure to sunshine. They lived in inner cities in over-crowded congested dwellings with narrow alleys. Prolonged winters as well as pollution from burning coal and wood further decreased sunrays from reaching the Earth, causing severe deficiency of vitamin D. Children were particularly affected as their developing bones suffered severely from the consequences of vitamin D deficiency. Moving like a shadow across the land, rickets erupted in Northeastern U.S. as big industrial cities popped up in this country. By 1900, approximately 80% of children living in Boston suffered from rickets.

By the 1930's, the link between rickets and vitamin D deficiency was well established. This remarkable discovery led to the fortification of milk with vitamin D. In the countries which adopted this practice of vitamin D fortification, rickets was mostly eradicated.

With the elimination of rickets, medical science mostly *forgot* about vitamin D until a few decades ago when it was discovered that <u>vitamin D is really not a vitamin, but a hormone</u>.

What is a hormone? A hormone is a substance that is produced in one part of the body, enters the blood stream and exerts its effects at sites distant from the original site of its production. For example, thyroid hormone is produced in the thyroid gland. It then travels through the blood stream and exerts its actions on the heart, muscle, brain and almost every other organ in the body.

Vitamin D: a Hormone

Vitamin D is produced in the skin from 7-dehydrocholesterol (pro-vitamin D3) which is derived from cholesterol. Here is evidence that cholesterol is not all bad, contrary to what most people think these days. The fact is that cholesterol is a precursor for most hormones in your body.

Type B Ultraviolet rays (UVB) from the sun act on pro-vitamin D3 and convert it into pre-vitamin D3, which is then converted into vitamin D3. Medically speaking, we call it cholecalciferol. Vitamin D3 then leaves the skin and gets into the blood stream where it is carried on a special protein called a vitamin D-binding protein.

Through blood circulation, vitamin D3 reaches various organs in the body. In the liver, vitamin D3 undergoes a slight change in its chemical structure. At that point, it is called 25, hydroxy cholecalciferol or 25 (OH) Vitamin D3 (or calcifediol). It is then carried through the blood stream to the kidneys where it goes through another change in its chemical structure. At that point, it is called 1,25 dihydroxy cholecalciferol or 1,25 $(OH)_2$ Vitamin D3 (or calcitriol). This is the active form of vitamin D. It gets in the blood stream and goes to various parts of the body and exerts its actions. Now you understand why vitaminD is really a hormone.

With the discovery that vitamin D is a hormone, scientists found the main effect of vitamin D was on calcium and phosphorus absorption from the intestines.

It was also realized that people with kidney failure cannot adequately convert 25 (OH) vitamin D into 1,25 $(OH)_2$ vitamin D. Therefore, people with chronic kidney failure on dialysis were placed on a synthetic supplement of 1,25 $(OH)_2$ vitamin D which is also called calcitriol. Drug companies saw an opportunity and started manufacturing calcitriol (brand name Rocaltrol). Soon, it became a standard of medical practice to prescribe calcitriol to every patient on chronic kidney dialysis. *For most physicians, this is where their knowledge of vitamin D ends.*

In the last couple of decades, researchers discovered that vitamin D is not only involved in the absorption of calcium and phosphorus from the intestines, but also plays an important role in the normal functioning of *every system* in the body, as I discussed earlier in Chapter 1.

Scientists also discovered that vitamin D deficiency is much more prevalent than was previously thought. In fact, it has reached epidemic proportions. This may partly explain the epidemics of chronic fatigue, osteoporosis, heart disease, hypertension, diabetes, cancer, asthma and other immunologic diseases. Proper vitamin D supplementation may help to prevent as well as treat most of these medical diseases.

CHAPTER 3

Misconceptions About Vitamin D

There are a lot of misconceptions about vitamin D. Here are some common ones I've heard:

- "I drink milk, so I can't be low in vitamin D."
- "I take a multivitamin and a calcium supplement every day, so my vitamin D should be okay."
- "I eat healthy, so my vitamin D should be fine."
- "I play tennis outdoors twice a week. How can I be low in vitamin D?"
- "I don't want to take vitamin D because I read about vitamin D toxicity. It's quite scary."
- "I'm outdoors at least 15 minutes a day. My vitamin D should be fine."
- "I live in sunny California. How can I be low in Vitamin D?"

When people make these comments, I simply advise them to have their vitamin D level checked. They're often surprised at the results. Most people turn out to be low in vitamin D.

Contrary to common belief, milk is a poor source of vitamin D. In the U.S., one cup of milk contains 100 I.U. of vitamin D. Now imagine trying to drink about 20 cups of milk a day to get a good level of vitamin D! The usual cup of milk added to your cereal provides you with just a miniscule amount of vitamin D.

People who take multivitamins and calcium supplements are under the impression they get enough vitamin D. Not true! I check vitamin D level in my patients who are on multivitamins and calcium supplements. Almost all of them turn out to be low in vitamin D. Why?

At the root of the problem is the recommended daily dose of vitamin D, which is old and outdated. Currently, the recommended daily dose of vitamin D is 200 - 600 I.U. (International Units). This dose of vitamin D was developed to prevent rickets, a bone disease in children.

In the last decade, scientific studies have shown that vitamin D is not only important for the health of bones, but is vital for the health of virtually every cell in the body. However, you need a much higher dose of vitamin D than 200 - 600 I.U. a day to achieve these results.

In contrast, multivitamins and calcium supplements continue to follow the recommended daily dose. So when you read the label of a multivitamin or a calcium supplement, which claims that it meets 100% of the daily requirement for vitamin D, you obviously assume you take the right amounts of vitamin D. However, if you have your vitamin D level checked, you'll be in for a big surprise. Your vitamin D level will likely be low.

Sunshine is an excellent source of vitamin D. However, playing tennis or golf a couple of times a week is not enough. Neither is taking a walk 3 times a week or spending some weekends outdoors. I am amazed to see articles on vitamin D deficiency in newspapers and magazines which recommend that outdoor sun exposure for 15 minutes a day is enough to take care of your vitamin D requirement. How inaccurate!

For the last 10 years, I have checked vitamin D levels in my patients. Many of these people are active - outdoors about 30 to 60 minutes a day, playing golf or other sports two to three times a week and walking three times a week. They take multivitamins and calcium supplements containing vitamin D and yet they are still quite low in vitamin D. This is reality!

So why do people have these misconceptions about vitamin D? To answer this question, you have to answer another question. Where do people get their medical information? Usually from newspapers, magazines, TV and the internet. Doctors are too busy to sit down and educate their patients, especially on a subject like vitamins. People are left to the mercy of information provided by the news media. Unfortunately, many articles are written by people who have no medical experience. Many of these professional writers simply gather information on vitamin D from previously published articles. In this way, inaccurate information in those previous articles simply gets recycled.

CHAPTER 4

Natural Sources of Vitamin D

Where do we get our vitamin D? A lot of people recognize that we get vitamin D from the sun: Vitamin D is the "sunshine" vitamin. But are we getting enough vitamin D from the sun?

Sun

The Sun is the major source of vitamin D. How much vitamin D you get from the sun varies from person to person. There are a number of factors that determine the amount of vitamin D you can get from the sun.

1. Geographic Location.

Where you live determines how much vitamin D you can get from the sun. The farther North you live from the equator, the less is the intensity of sun rays reaching the earth. Therefore, your skin forms less vitamin D if you live in northern climates such as the North Eastern U.S., Canada and northern European countries.

2. Season and time of the day.

Your skin can form more vitamin D during summer, but less during winter. This is because fewer sun rays reach the surface of Earth during winter. Similarly, the best time for the synthesis of vitamin D is between 10 am and 3 pm.

3. Sun Screens, Pollution, Shade, Glass Windows, Clothing

Sunscreens, pollution, shade, glass windows and clothing all decrease the amount of UVB rays entering your skin and therefore, reduce the normal production of vitamin D by the skin. A sunscreen with a Sun Protection Factor (SPF) of 8 or more reduces the ability of the skin to form vitamin D by more than 95%. Complete cloud cover, shade and severe pollution reduces solar UVB energy by 50%.

4. Age

Compared to a young person, the skin of an elderly person contains much less 7-dehydrocholesterol. Therefore, the skin of an elderly person typically manufactures only about 25% of vitamin D3 as compared to the skin of a young person.

5. Color of skin

The color of your skin comes from a pigment in the skin called melanin. The more melanin you have, the darker your skin color. Melanin serves as a natural sun screen and blocks sunrays from getting into deeper layers of skin. Therefore, darker skin is less efficient in synthesizing vitamin D from the sun as compared to fair skin. For example, an African American person may need more than 10 fold the time in the sun as compared to a white person in order to produce the same amount of vitamin D. However, people with darker skin are less likely to get skin cancer due to the protective effects of melanin. Nature is such an equalizer!

Diet ━━━━━━━━━━━━━━━━━━━━━━━━

Diet is not a major source of vitamin D. Some food items that naturally contain small amounts of vitamin D include oily fish such as salmon, mackerel and blue fish. The amount of vitamin D in fish remains unchanged if it is baked, but decreases about 50% if fish is fried. Also, farm raised salmon has only about 25% of vitamin D compared to wild salmon.

Vitamin D is also present in small quantities in vegetables, meat and egg yolk. Natural milk does not contain vitamin D, but most milk in the U.S. is fortified with vitamin D and therefore, contains small amounts of vitamin D. Vitamin D is also added in small amounts in dairy products such as cheese and some yogurts.

Most cereals in the U.S. are also fortified with small amounts of vitamin D. Orange juice is also fortified with a small amount of vitamin D.

The following food items are supposed to contain the indicated amount of vitamin D:

- Salmon, cooked (3.5 ounces) 360, I.U.
- Mackerel, cooked (3.5 ounces) 345, I.U.
- Canned Tuna (3.0 ounces) 200, I.U.
- Sardines canned in oil, drained (1.75 ounces) 250, I.U.
- Raw Shiitake Mushrooms (10 ounces) 76, I.U.
- Fortified Milk, one cup (8 ounces or 240 ml) 100, I.U.
- Fortified Orange Juice, one cup (8 ounces or 240 ml) 100, I.U.
- Fortified Cereal 40-80 I.U. per serving.
- Egg, 1 whole (vitamin D is found in the yolk) 20, I.U.
- Liver of beef, cooked (3.5 ounces) 15, I.U.
- Swiss cheese (1 ounce) 12, I.U.

* I.U. = International Units

A word of caution! You can't rely on the stated quantities of vitamin D on food labels. In one study (1), researchers found that vitamin D in milk was less than 80% of the stated amount. The vitamin D content of fish is highly variable.

Vitamin D3 versus Vitamin D2 ────────────

Natural vitamin D comes in two forms: vitamin D3 and vitamin D2. The proper chemical name for vitamin D3 is cholecalciferol and vitamin D2 is ergocalciferol. Vitamin D from the sun and fatty fish is vitamin D3 (cholecalciferol) and the one from vegetables is Vitamin D2 (ergocalciferol).

Over the counter vitamin supplements are mostly vitamin D3. A prescription form of vitamin D has been vitamin D2 which comes in a large dose of 50,000 I.U. Recently, vitamin D3 has also become available in a high dose of 50,000 I.U.

Some studies (2) have suggested that vitamin D3 is superior to vitamin D2, but a recent study (3) suggested that vitamin D2 is as good as vitamin D3.

In my clinical practice, I find both vitamin D3 and vitamin D2 to be effective. I primarily use vitamin D3 in most patients who are mild to moderately low in vitamin D. I have been using vitamin D2 in those patients who are severely deficient in vitamin D and need heavy doses to build up their vitamin D stores. After building up stores of vitamin D, I switch them from vitamin D2 to vitamin D3. Now that vitamin D3 is available in large doses of 50,000 I.U., I will start using it even in severe cases of vitamin D deficiency.

REFERENCES:

1. Holick MF, Shao Q, Liu WW, et al. The vitamin D content of fortified milk and infant formula. *N Engl J Med.* 1992;326(18):1178-81.
2. Armas LA, Hollis BW, Heaney RP. Vitamin D2 is much less effective than vitamin D3 in humans. *J Clin Endocrinol Metab.* 2004;89 (11)5387-91.
3. Holick MF, Biancuzzo RM, Chen TC et al. Vitamin D2 is as effective as vitamin D3 in maintaining circulating concentrations of 25 (OH) vitamin D. *J Clin Endocrinol Metab.* 2008;93(3):677-81.

CHAPTER 5

An Epidemic of Vitamin D Deficiency

Believe it or not, there's an epidemic of vitamin D deficiency! Ten years ago, I started investigating vitamin D levels in my patients. To my surprise, the vast majority turned out to be low in Vitamin D. My experience is in line with other researchers.

For example, researchers recently analyzed the data on vitamin D status in the U.S. adult population from the 2000-2004 National Health and Nutrition Examination Survey (NHANES) (1). They were amazed to discover that 50-78% of Americans were low in vitamin D. What's alarming is that the situation is getting worse. Vitamin D levels in Americans were found to be lower during the 2000-2004 period compared to the 1988-1994 period (2). Clearly vitamin D deficiency is getting out of control.

Not only Americans, but people all around the world are suffering from vitamin D deficiency. For example, in the United Kingdom, 90% of adults were found to be low in vitamin D according to the nationally representative data collected between 1992 and 2001 (3).

Vitamin D deficiency is the true epidemic of our times. It is perhaps more common than any other medical condition at the present time.

It spares no age. ▬▬▬▬▬▬▬▬▬▬▬▬▬▬▬▬▬▬

Infants, children, adults and elderly are all low in vitamin D. In my extensive clinical experience, it's rare to find someone who has a good level of vitamin D. In my practice, the age of patients range from 15 to 95. I find an overwhelming majority of these patients to be low in vitamin D. Several studies have clearly demonstrated that vitamin D deficiency spans across all age groups.

It spares no geographic location. ▬▬▬▬▬▬▬▬

According to the old paradigm, vitamin D deficiency exists only in northern areas with severe prolonged winters such as Canada, the Northeastern U.S., the U.K. and other northern European countries. However, in reality, vitamin D deficiency is prevalent even in sunny, warm places such as the Middle East, India, Pakistan, New Zealand and Australia. In my own extensive clinical experience in southern California, I have found that most of my patients are low in vitamin D. Vitamin D deficiency is a global phenomenon.

If you live in northern climates, you are even more prone to vitamin D deficiency because you can't get enough vitamin D during winter months. In places above 42 degrees North latitude (approximately a line drawn between the northern border of California and Boston), there isn't sufficient solar UVB (Ultra Violet B) energy to form vitamin D in the skin during winter time (from November through February). In far northern latitudes, this decrease in solar energy may last up to 6 months.

In areas below 34 degrees North latitude (approximately a line drawn between Los Angeles and Columbia, North Carolina), there's enough solar UVB energy for skin synthesis of vitamin D throughout the year. But even in these areas, the sun can't give you vitamin D if you avoid it by using clothing, sun screen lotions or by simply staying out of it. Therefore, you may live in a sunny place south of 34 degrees latitude, but still be low in vitamin D.

Several clinical studies have shown that vitamin D deficiency is extremely common in the sunny Middle East, primarily because the skin doesn't get enough sun exposure. Due to cultural habits, people avoid the sun and cover most of their body with clothes. This is particularly true in the case of women living in these countries.

It spares no race.

Although darker skin is less efficient in synthesizing vitamin D from sun exposure as compared to fair skin, people with fair skin avoid the sun more than people with dark skin for fear of skin cancer. In my extensive clinical experience, I've found people from various racial and ethnic groups to be low in vitamin D.

What are the Causes for the Epidemic of Vitamin D Deficiency?

1. Modern Life-Style

Let's take a historic look on vitamin D. It appears that humans started their journey on planet Earth in Africa where there was plenty of sunshine. With slow migration northwards over thousands of years, the skin gradually adapted to colder northern climates by reducing the content of its natural sun screen (melanin) and consequently, skin became lighter in color. People with light skin were then able to synthesize enough vitamin D in brief exposures to sunshine.

Vitamin D deficiency is a relatively new phenomenon. Scientists first recognized it in the seventeenth century in the U.K. and other Northern European countries. Interestingly, it coincided with the period of the Industrial Revolution when people flocked to big industrial cities such as London and Warsaw and lived in multistoried buildings with narrow, dark alleys. Pollution from coal burning factories created a thick layer of smog. These factors significantly reduced the amount of sun rays reaching Earth in these regions which already had marginal sunshine during long winter periods.

The phenomenon of the Industrial Revolution continued in the newly discovered lands of America and Canada. In addition, native Africans were enslaved and transported in ships to America over a period of months. Compare this rapid migration to the thousands of years it took for early Africans to migrate to Europe, allowing for their skin to adapt to less sunshine. In contrast, this recent migration was extraordinarily rapid, allowing no time for the skin to adapt to conditions of less sunshine. For this reason, African-Americans as a group are particularly low in vitamin D.

In recent years, worldwide migration happens at an even faster pace. In a matter of hours, you can migrate from one region of the world to another. That's why people from India and Pakistan who migrate to the U.K. and North America are particularly low in vitamin D.

Now consider another interesting phenomenon. As a result of the Industrial Revolution, people with fair skin were able to rapidly migrate to Southern regions with plenty of sunshine. Their skin didn't have time to adapt to these new sunny environments. Therefore, these fair skinned people started developing skin cancer from excessive sun exposure. This led to the development of sunscreen lotions and the drum beat of "avoid the sun!" Even people with dark skin started applying sunscreen lotions under the impression that "it's a healthy habit."

The main reason we're facing an epidemic of vitamin D deficiency is our modern life-style, which minimizes our exposure to the sun. Technological revolution has dramatically changed lifestyles around the globe. Most people work indoors. They leave their homes early in the morning and return home around sunset or even after dark (especially during winter time). Even at lunch, most people drive to a restaurant or stay inside to eat. Many people spend their lunch break in their office. Over the weekend, we watch TV or surf the internet for entertainment. Teenagers usually stay indoors hooked to a computer or playing video games rather than going outdoors and playing real sports. While shopping, people are mostly indoors thanks to huge grocery stores and shopping malls. Many of the elderly live in assisted living facilities or nursing homes and don't get any sun exposure.

Just observe yourself. How often do you, your family and friends stay indoors while carrying out usual activities of daily living?

2. Sun Phobia

Over the last 30 years or so, sun avoidance has been successfully drilled into the minds of the general public. People are simply scared of the ill-effects of the sun such as skin cancer, wrinkles and aging spots.

Due to sun phobia, people avoid sun exposure at all costs. When we go outside for even a little while, we make sure to apply sun screen. Parents compulsively apply sunscreen before they allow their children to go outdoors. Many people don't realize that sunscreen also prevents vitamin D synthesis in the skin.

3. Obesity

Vitamin D is fat soluble. Therefore, it gets stored in the fat in your body. In obese individuals, there is excessive storage of vitamin D in fat. Consequently, the circulating level of vitamin D is low in these individuals.

Obesity has reached epidemic proportions in the U.S. and the rest of the world is also catching up in this regard. The epidemic of obesity is contributing to the epidemic of vitamin D deficiency. It's interesting to note that in most cases, obesity is a product of our modern life-style as well.

4. Medical Illnesses
A. Malabsorption:
Because vitamin D is fat soluble, vitamin D deficiency can

develop in medical conditions that cause malabsorption of fat, such as surgical resection of the small intestine and stomach, chronic pancreatitis, pancreatic surgery, celiac sprue, Crohn's colitis and cystic fibrosis.

B. Liver and Kidney Diseases:

Vitamin D from the blood is taken up by the liver where it is transformed into 25 (OH) Vitamin D which in the kidneys, is further transformed into 1,25 $(OH)_2$ Vitamin D. Therefore, vitamin D deficiency develops in chronic liver disease such as cirrhosis and in chronic kidney disease.

5. Medications

Some medications can further decrease vitamin D level. These medications include:

- Phenytoin (brand name Dilatin)
- Phenobarbital
- Rifampin
- Orlistat (brand names Xenical and Alli)
- Cholestyramine (brand names Questran, LoCholest and Prevalite)
- Steroids

*Steroids, in particular can cause a severe deficiency of vitamin D.

I often see patients who have been on these drugs for a long time, yet they're completely unaware these drugs can rob them of vitamin D. They react with disbelief when I inform them about the relationship between these medications and vitamin D deficiency. "Why didn't my other doctor tell me about it?" is their usual question. Of course, it's your doctor's responsibility to inform you about the side-effects of medicines. Unfortunately, the reality is that some do and some don't. So educate yourself and be a partner in taking charge of your health. That's why you're reading this book. Nothing can be more rewarding for me than providing you with the information you need to help take care of your vitamin D needs in collaboration with your health care provider.

6. Flaws with the Current Recommendations on Vitamin D Intake.

Many people taking vitamins assume that their vitamin D level is okay because the label on their vitamin bottle says it meets 100% of the daily requirements. This misconception is one of the major reasons for vitamin D deficiency among those people who are proactive in taking care of their health.

Vitamin manufacturers follow government guidelines for the daily recommended amounts of various vitamins and minerals. As of 2009, the recommended daily allowance of vitamin D in the U.S. is: 200 I.U. (International Units) from birth to age 50, 400 I.U. from age 50 to 70 and 600 I.U. if you are older than 70.

Most researchers in the field of vitamin D (myself included) find these recommendations for vitamin D to be inadequate. In a review article published in the July 2006 issue of the *American Journal of Clinical Nutrition*, the authors concluded that for most people, the optimal level of vitamin D is not attainable with the currently recommended daily allowances of vitamin D (4). In March 2007, a number of researchers published an editorial urging a change in the recommendations on daily intake of vitamin D to 1700 I.U. in order to obtain a desirable blood concentration of vitamin D (5).

REFERENCES:
1. Yetley EA, Assessing vitamin D status of the U.S. population. *Am J Clin Nutr.* 2008;88(2)558S-564S.
2. Ginde AA, Liu MC, Camargo CA Jr. Demographic differences and trends of vitamin D insufficiency in the US population, 1988-2004. *Arch Intern Med.* 2009;169(6):626-632.
3. Prentice A. Vitamin D deficiency: a global perspective. *Nutr Rev.* 2008; 66(10 suppl 2): S153-164.

4. Bischoff-Ferrari H et al. Current recommended vitamin D may not be optimal. *Am J Clin Nutr*. 2006; 84:18-28.

5. Vieth R, Bischoff-Ferrari H, Boucher BJ, Dawson- Hughes B, Garland CF, Heaney RP, et al. The urgent need to recommend an intake of vitamin D that is effective. *Am J Clin Nutr* 2007; 85:649-50.

CHAPTER 6

Vitamin D Deficiency and Body Aches, Pains and Chronic Fatigue Syndrome

Body aches, pains and chronic fatigue are the most common complaints that doctors hear from their patients. While there are many reasons why people develop body aches, pains and fatigue, one *common and easily treatable* cause is vitamin D deficiency. Unfortunately, it often remains undiagnosed and untreated. Consequently, people continue to suffer from chronic pains and fatigue for many years.

The Link Between Vitamin D Deficiency and Body Aches, Pains and Chronic Fatigue

Vitamin D has a close relationship with another hormone known as Parathyroid Hormone (PTH) which is produced by the parathyroid glands, four tiny structures lying low in the neck behind the thyroid gland.

Under normal conditions, PTH is important in maintaining a normal level of calcium in the blood, which is important for the normal functioning of each and every cell in the body, particularly muscle cells and heart cells. PTH maintains a normal level of calcium in the blood by acting on the kidneys, bones and intestines. By acting on the kidneys, it prevents excessive loss of calcium in the urine. It also helps the kidneys convert 25 (OH) vitamin D into 1, 25 $(OH)_2$ vitamin D, which then acts on the intestines and helps in the absorption of calcium and phosphorus into the blood stream. By acting on the bones, PTH dissolves their calcium and brings that calcium into the blood stream.

In people with vitamin D deficiency, the parathyroid glands start to produce more than the normal amount of PTH. Large amounts of PTH then cause excessive dissolving of calcium from the bones. Consequently, bones become weak. These people then start experiencing bone aches and pains, which are diffuse and deep. People often can't describe them precisely, but say things like:

"Doc, my whole body hurts."

"It hurts all over."

"My body just aches. I feel like someone pulled the plug."

But sometimes, patients can describe these pains with precision: "Doc, this pain feels deep, as if my bones are aching."

As a result of generalized aches and pains, you also feel tired and fatigued. You may feel like taking a nap in the afternoon.

Typically, you visit your family physician who puts you on pain medications and runs a bunch of expensive tests, which often turn out to be normal. You are then referred to a number of specialists who order more special diagnostic tests. Results of all these tests are often normal as well. Meanwhile, no one orders a test for vitamin D and PTH and therefore, your true diagnosis remains elusive.

Some specialist may give you the diagnosis of Fibromyalgia, Chronic Pain Syndrome or Chronic Fatigue Syndrome. This simply describes your symptoms in fancy medical terminology, but obviously doesn't get to the root of your problem.

You and your physician are perplexed. What's really causing these pains? "It must be in your head." Your doctor suggests an anti-anxiety / anti-depression medication. You may actually be anxious and/or depressed because of your frustration. After all, you've undergone extensive testing and yet no one really knows what's wrong with you. You start thinking the worst: "Maybe it's some cancer they haven't diagnosed yet." It's understandable if you're anxious or depressed.

By this time, you're willing to accept any diagnosis. So you buy into any explanation your physician offers. I have heard all kinds of interesting explanations given to patients by their physicians. Here are some examples:

"Your aches and pains are due to anxiety and depression."
"It's just from getting old!"
"You have Fibromyalgia."
"You have Chronic Fatigue Syndrome"
"You're suffering from frailty."

So your physician puts you on anti-anxiety/anti-depression medications in addition to the pain killers you're already taking. Each drug may cause some side-effects. Often you develop new symptoms for which you're given a new medication and then you experience their side-effects. A vicious cycle sets in.

Before you know it, you're on a long list of medications and still having a lot of symptoms, including generalized aches and pains. Because these medications give temporary relief of your symptoms, you get attached to them. You start to think you can't live without them. You go from physician to physician looking for pain killers and anti-anxiety medications, which sooner or later, they refuse to refill. Eventually, you may be referred to a pain specialist. Now you are in for some heavy duty pain medications and sometimes, your pain specialist recommends complicated procedures aimed at treating your Chronic Pain Syndrome. These pain medications are often narcotics with potential for addiction and many other serious side-effects. Over the years, I have seen many such unfortunate messed up cases.

In medical literature, there are several studies which clearly demonstrate that patients with chronic muscle aches and pains continue to suffer simply because their physicians fail to diagnose vitamin D deficiency as the root cause of their symptoms. In one such study (1), researchers investigated vitamin D level in patients with chronic muscle aches and pains at a university-affiliated clinic in Minneapolis, Minnesota. They were amazed to find out that nearly all of these patients were low in vitamin D. Many had *severe* deficiency of vitamin D. Some had been seeing doctors for years and vitamin D deficiency was not even considered as a cause of their disabling symptoms.

Perhaps now you realize how frequently physicians miss the diagnosis of vitamin D deficiency as the root cause of chronic muscle aches and pains. Therefore, you have to be proactive in taking charge of your health. Get your vitamin D level tested and get on the proper dose of Vitamin D! (see Chapters 22 and 23 on Diagnosis and Treatment of vitamin D deficiency) I have many patients in my practice whose body aches and pains simply disappeared after proper replacement of vitamin D.

Secondary hyperparathyroidism ▬▬▬▬▬▬▬▬▬▬▬

When vitamin D deficiency goes undiagnosed and untreated, PTH level in the blood becomes elevated. In medical terms, we call it *secondary hyperparathyroidism*. Your blood calcium level is normal at this stage of your disease of chronic vitamin D deficiency. Physicians generally don't order a PTH test when your calcium level is normal. That's what they were taught in medical schools! Therefore, secondary hyperparathyroidism often remains undiagnosed.

Unfortunately, this high level of PTH comes with a price. It erodes your bones causing them to ache. Medically speaking, we call it osteomalacia. In plain language, your bones are weak, they ache and they can also easily fracture.

Tertiary Hyperparathyroidism / Primary Hyperparathyroidism ▬▬

If vitamin D deficiency and resulting secondary hyperparathyroidism is not properly treated, eventually, one or more of your parathyroid glands may get enlarged from all the overwork they have to do. At this stage of chronic vitamin D deficiency, your *blood calcium level also becomes elevated*. I call this advanced stage of chronic vitamin D deficiency *tertiary hyperparathyroidism*. Tertiary means that your disease has progressed from secondary hyperparathyroidism to a more advanced stage. But, traditionally, it is called *primary hyperparathyroidism*.

Typically, a physician is trained to order a blood level of PTH in a patient with elevated calcium level in the blood. If PTH turns out to be high, the patient is diagnosed with primary hyperparathyroidism. As a knee jerk reflex, the patient is then sent for parathyroid surgery.

I have a problem with this terminology of primary hyperparathyroidism because it implies that your PTH level became elevated for no obvious reason. With this mind set, physicians, even at this advanced stage of the disease, don't order a vitamin D level. This terminology of primary hyperparathyroidism comes from the era when we did not test our patients for vitamin D deficiency as we do now.

My belief is that most cases of primary hyperparathyroidism are actually tertiary hyperparathyroidism, the result of years and years of untreated vitamin D deficiency. It's interesting to note that the prevalence of primary hyperparathyroidism has increased tremendously in the last three decades. This precisely coincides with the widespread usage of sunscreen lotions, and an epidemic of obesity both of which have contributed to the epidemic of vitamin D deficiency.

CASE STUDY

Bob is a 51 year old Caucasian gentleman who consulted me after he saw several specialists for slightly elevated calcium level in the blood. His calcium was staying between 10.5 to 11 mg/dl (with normal being less than 10.5 mg/dl). His PTH level was also elevated at 111 pg/ml. (with a normal range of 10-65). He was diagnosed with primary hyperparathyroidism and as a knee jerk reflex, his specialist recommended parathyroid surgery.

No one checked Bob's vitamin D level. He had chronic low back pain. His bone density test showed that bones in his lumber spine were quite weakened to the point of being diagnosed with osteoporosis. At this juncture, he came to see me.

I ordered his vitamin D level which turned out to be quite low. I placed him on Vitamin D3, initially 2000 I.U. a day and then increased to 3000 I.U. a day. To everyone's surprise, his blood calcium came down into the normal range as his vitamin D level got to the optimal level. At the same time, his PTH level also came down to normal.

Why did his blood calcium come down instead of going up on high doses of vitamin D, as most physicians would have expected? **Because his PTH level came down.** *PTH is a very potent hormone for increasing blood calcium level: It does so by increasing calcium absorption from the intestines, by decreasing calcium loss in the urine and by dissolving calcium from the bones. So, when PTH level* comes down, so does the calcium level.

Bob's low back pain resolved and his bone density improved as his PTH level came down. Bob has been under my care for 4 years and his calcium, vitamin D and PTH levels have remained normal.

This case clearly shows how vitamin D deficiency can cause an elevation in PTH level (secondary hyperparathyroidism), osteoporosis, body aches and pains and in time, even an increase in blood calcium level (tertiary hyperparathyroidism, which is traditionally termed as primary hyperparathyroidism). Treating the root cause, vitamin D deficiency, with large doses of vitamin D is the appropriate treatment. With the correct diagnosis and treatment, Bob fortunately avoided parathyroid surgery.

When to Consider Parathyroid Surgery ━━━━━━

In this late stage of parathyroid disease (tertiary or primary hyperparathyroidism) due to chronic vitamin D deficiency, if your blood calcium remains elevated above 11 mg/dl even after you have achieved an optimal blood level of vitamin D (discussed in Chapter 23 on Treatment of Vitamin D deficiency), you should consider parathyroid surgery.

Some people with elevated blood calcium level may also develop kidney stones. These patients should have parathyroid surgery. High calcium in the blood leads to high spillage of calcium in the urine and consequently, increases your risk for calcium stone formation in the kidneys. This high spillage of calcium in the urine can be easily diagnosed with a test ordered by your physician. In this test, called 24 hours urine for calcium, you collect your urine for 24 hours and take it to the laboratory for calcium testing. Contact the laboratory in advance for special instructions as well as a special bottle to collect your urine.

If you have high blood calcium, high PTH level and your 24 hours urine calcium is more than 300 mg, you are at high risk for calcium stone formation in the kidneys. You may consider parathyroid surgery even if you don't yet have kidney stones.

Some patients with tertiary (primary) hyperparathyroidism may develop severe osteoporosis and are at risk for fracture of their bones. They should also consider parathyroid surgery.

You Need Vitamin D Replacement Even After Parathyroid Surgery. ▬

Parathyroid surgery does not treat vitamin D deficiency. Symptoms of vitamin D deficiency such as body aches, pains and chronic fatigue are not going to go away just by doing parathyroid surgery. Many physicians are not aware of this fact. Typically, patients undergo parathyroid surgery, but still no one orders vitamin D level. Please remember that even after parathyroid surgery, you will need proper replacement with vitamin D.

CASE STUDY

Evelyn, a 62 year old female, started having generalized body aches and pains. She saw her family physician who referred her to a specialist at a prestigious medical clinic. She was told that she had elevated PTH level and was advised to undergo surgery on her parathyroid glands. She agreed and underwent surgery.

After surgery, her symptoms didn't improve and actually got worse. Obviously, she was quite frustrated. "I hurt all over Doc! The kind of pain that never goes away. It's deep in my bones. Nothing has helped. Not even parathyroid surgery. I don't think I am going to make it. " I vividly remember her

---

utter frustration when she came to see me.

I ordered her vitamin D level, which was very low. I placed her on the proper dose of vitamin D. To her astonishment, her symptoms that haunted her for years simply went away. Now she pursues a joyful, active life and is obviously a big believer in vitamin D supplementation.

Perhaps now you can understand why an early diagnosis and proper treatment of vitamin D deficiency can save you from a lot of misery. You can prevent body aches, pains, osteoporosis, kidney stones and parathyroid surgery.

REFERENCES:

1. Plotnikoff GA, Quigley JM. Prevalence of severe hypovitaminosis D in patients with persistent, nonspecific musculoskeletal pain. Mayo Clin Proc. 2003;(78):1463-1470.

CHAPTER 7

Vitamin D Deficiency and Osteoporosis

What is Osteoporosis?

In simple terms, osteoporosis means "weak bones." That places you at increased risk of breaking a bone even after a trivial trauma that otherwise wouldn't cause a fracture.

Diagnosis of Osteoporosis

The most commonly used test to diagnose osteoporosis is called Bone DXA (Dual X-rays Absorptiometry). It's like getting an X-ray and only takes about 15 minutes. The test uses X-rays, but in a very small amount. The test is usually done at the hip and lower back (lumbar spine). Sometimes, it is also done at the forearm.

A much less frequently used test is called Quantitative CT scan of the spine. Exposure to X-ray radiation is much higher in this test compared to the bone DXA test.

Sometimes, an ultrasound is also used to screen people for osteoporosis, but results of an ultrasound should be confirmed with a bone DXA.

All of these tests measure your bone mineral density (BMD). In reports of the bone DXA test, you get a number called T-score.

This T-score is obtained by comparing your bone density to the average bone density of young people from data stored in the machine. In this way, we guess your bone density from when you were young. Scientifically speaking, this isn't very accurate, but it's all we have to work with.

Normal T-score is above -1 SD (Standard Deviation). If your T score is between -1 and   -2.5 SD, your diagnosis is osteopenia, and if this score is at -2.5 or below, your diagnosis is osteoporosis. In other words, osteopenia is a mild, early stage of weakening of bones and osteoporosis is a more advanced stage.

Who Gets Osteoporosis?

While no one is immune, the following medical conditions increase your risk for Osteopenia/Osteoporosis:
- Vitamin D deficiency
- Elderly men and women
- Post-menopausal women
- Men with low testosterone
- Patients on steroids
- Patients with an over-active thyroid gland
- Patients who receive too much thyroid hormone in a pill form
- Patients with Diabetes
- Patients with Rheumatoid arthritis

The Relationship Between Vitamin D Deficiency and Osteoporosis

In medical literature, it's well established that vitamin D deficiency is a major cause for osteoporosis. A number of studies have clearly shown that people with osteoporosis are often low in vitamin D. In one such study (1), researchers looked at the bone mineral density, calcium intake and vitamin D level of 4958 women and 5003 men living in the U.S.; They found that there was a direct correlation between vitamin D level and bone mineral density: the lower the vitamin D level, the lower the bone mineral density and the higher the vitamin D level, the higher the bone mineral density.

In the same study, researchers also found that calcium intake of more than about 600 mg per day did not cause any increase in bone mineral density in the majority of patients. This obviously contradicts the standard advice to take at least 1500 mg per day of calcium to keep your bones healthy. It's clear that vitamin D plays the predominant role in determining bone strength. Calcium intake of about 600 mg per day is adequate if you have a good level of vitamin D.

In another study (2), researchers obtained vitamin D levels in 1292 menopausal women with osteopenia or osteoporosis living in France. They found that 90% of these women were low in vitamin D.

The main reason of concern regarding low bone mineral density is that if you have osteopenia or osteoporosis, it increases your risk for fracturing a bone. When you have osteoporosis, even a trivial trauma can cause a fracture.

Is there a direct correlation between the level of vitamin D and risk for fracture? The answer is Yes. In an interesting study (3), researchers investigated the hypothesis that low vitamin D places you at risk for a fracture of the bone, regardless of whether the trauma is trivial or heavy. The research was carried out at a hospital in New York. The researchers found that 59% of all patients (men and women) with a bone fracture after any degree of trauma were low in vitamin D. Even more impressive was the finding that up to 80% of women who sustained a fracture after a trivial or heavy trauma were low in vitamin D.

Treatment of Osteopenia/Osteoporosis ━━━━━━━━

When you're low in vitamin D, as most people are, your bones start to weaken. Therefore, the first step in the treatment of osteopenia and osteoporosis is to achieve a good level of vitamin D in your body. As discussed in Chapter 23, Treatment of Vitamin D Deficiency, for most people that means taking a large dose of Vitamin D supplement.

CASE STUDY

Lisa, a 62 year old Caucasian female, consulted me for a number of symptoms including foot cramps. On her Bone DXA, she had a T-score of -2.2 SD at her lumbar spine and -1.7 SD at her hip. I diagnosed her with osteopenia and placed her on vitamin D3, 1000 I.U. a day. On this dose of vitamin D her 25 (OH) Vitamin D level was 34 ng/ml, which still was not optimal. So I increased her daily dose of vitamin D to 2000 I.U. a day.

Three years later, we repeated her bone DXA which showed a significant improvement in her T-scores: Now her T-score at her lumbar spine was -1.2 SD and at her hip it was -1.4 SD. This meant a 13% increase in her bone mineral density at the lumbar spine and a 5% increase in her bone mineral density at the hip. She was thrilled to see this kind of result with vitamin D supplementation alone. She no longer has any cramps in her feet either.

Unfortunately most physicians don't check vitamin D level in patients with osteopenia/osteoporosis and rush to prescription drugs. With this approach, vitamin D deficiency remains undiagnosed and untreated and can have serious health consequences.

CASE STUDY

At age 68, Charlotte was diagnosed with osteoporosis and placed on Fosamax (alendronate). Two years later, she fractured her left foot without any trauma and was taking a long time to heal. So her orthopedic surgeon referred her to me.

I found her 25 (OH) vitamin D to be 30 ng/ml (with a reference range of 9-54, it was obviously in the normal range), but I considered this level to be low. To confirm my clinical impression, I ordered a blood test for her parathyroid hormone (PTH) level which turned out to be elevated as 94 pg/ml (normal range 10-65), confirming that her vitamin D level was *low for her body* despite the normal range of her 25 (OH) vitamin D test. Her blood calcium was normal.

I diagnosed her with Secondary Hyperparathyroidism due to vitamin D deficiency (as discussed in Chapter 6) and placed her on vitamin D2, 50,000 I.U. weekly. In one month, her PTH came down to 74. Then the patient stopped taking her vitamin D for fear of vitamin D toxicity after reading an article in a newspaper. Two months later her PTH went up to 150 and she started having pain in her feet. I placed her back on vitamin D2, 50,000 I.U. weekly. Two months later, her PTH came down to 92. Then I switched her from vitamin D2 to vitamin D3, 2000 I.U. a day. Three months later, her PTH was down to 78. Over a period of several months, I increased her vitamin D3 intake to 8000 I.U. per day. At this high dose of vitamin D3, her most recent 25 (OH) vitamin D level was 77 ng/ml, and her PTH level was finally down to a normal level of 63 pg/ml.

In the last 4 years, proper vitamin D supplementation alone, without Fosamax (alendronate) or any other anti-osteoporosis drugs, has significantly improved her bone mineral density. Her recent T- score is -1.33 SD at the hip and -2.53 SD at the Lumbar spine. Compare it to her T-score of -1.4 SD at the hip and -3.03 SD at the lumbar spine before she got placed on Vitamin D. As you can see, there is a significant improvement in her T- score.

Charlotte feels great. No more fractures. No more foot pain.

Perhaps now you understand one of the most important factors causing osteopenia/osteoporosis is vitamin D deficiency. Unfortunately, it's often ignored. Meanwhile, pharmaceutical companies push their anti-osteoporosis drugs. Unfortunately, vitamin D doesn't have the backing and marketing muscle of a pharmaceutical company, because it's cheap and easily available over the counter. Physicians are taught to diagnose osteopenia or osteoporosis and prescribe a drug, without even checking vitamin D level. Sad, but it is a fact.

Over the years, I've seen many patients take expensive anti-osteoporosis drugs faithfully, but their osteoporosis gets worse. When checked, I find these patients to be quite low in vitamin D. Simply treating them with the right dose of vitamin D makes all the difference in the world.

CASE STUDY

Elizabeth was referred to me by her primary care physician. Her bone mineral density was deteriorating despite taking Actonel (risedronate). I tested her vitamin D level which turned out to be quite low. Her 25 (OH) vitamin D was 19 ng/ml. I added vitamin D3, 2000 I.U. a day. Her 25 (OH) vitamin D rose above 40 ng/ml and has stayed above 40 ng/ml for the last five years. Her last vitamin D level was 59 ng/ml. Over these last 5 years, her bone mineral density has improved. At age 78, Elizabeth feels great. In a letter to me she said, "What especially delights me is the return of my energy and zest for life. My family and friends have all commented on this and I owe many thanks to you."

Other researchers are also discovering what I have seen in my patients. In an excellent study (4), researchers from Belgium looked at the role of vitamin D in postmenopausal women who were taking anti-osteoporosis drugs. They divided these women into two groups: those with vitamin D deficiency and those with adequate vitamin D level. The researchers found that women with adequate vitamin D level had significantly more increase in their bone mineral density compared to women who had low vitamin D level. In addition, women with low vitamin D were at significantly high risk for fracture compared to women with adequate vitamin D level. Remember all of these women in both groups were on anti-osteoporosis drugs. To me, it's clear that *vitamin D is the most important factor in increasing your bone mineral density and preventing fractures.*

What osteoporosis really is and how anti-osteoporosis drugs work. ▬

Most people, including many doctors, don't quite understand what osteoporosis really is. Let me explain to you what really goes on in the bones when someone develops osteoporosis.

Bones, like every other organ in the body, are constantly going through a "death and birth cycle of tissues." Old bone is eaten away by specialized cells in the bone called osteoclasts. This process is called bone resorption. Then, another type of cells in the bones called osteoblasts lay down new bone in the space created by the resorption of the old bone. This process is called bone formation. These are slow processes and take place over a period of several months.

Bone resorption and bone formation are linked together: Bone resorption is followed by bone formation. One cannot happen without the other. They are tied together. In other words, for bone formation to take place, there has to be bone resorption. If bone resorption dwindles, so does bone formation.

Drugs to Treat Osteoporosis

The majority of drugs used to treat osteoporosis act by decreasing bone resorption. These drugs are called "Anti-resorptive drugs." These include the following drugs:

ANTI-RESORPTIVE DRUGS TO TREAT OSTEOPOROSIS

Brand Name	Generic Name
Fosamax	Alendronate
Actonel	Risedronate
Boniva	Ibandronate
Evista	Raloxifen
Miacalcin nasal spray	calcitonin

*Fosamax, Actonel and Boniva belong to the same family of drugs, which is called bisphosphonates.
*Estrogen replacement therapy also acts on bones as an anti-resorptive drug.

These "Anti-resorptive drugs" are primarily used to treat osteoporosis in post menopausal women because there is increased bone resorption in these women. These drugs slow down the resorption of bones, and therefore, can slow down bone loss. However, the downside of anti-resorptive drugs is that bone formation decreases as well, due to diminished bone resorption. Remember bone resorption and bone formation are interlinked.

Bone formation is further reduced if you don't have adequate levels of vitamin D in your blood. In this way, you can lose most of the gain in bone mineral density achieved through slowing down of bone resorption and end up with little or no improvement in your bone mineral density. If vitamin D deficiency is severe, your bone mineral density may actually decrease despite taking anti-resorptive drugs.

Therefore, it is absolutely crucial that you have a good level of vitamin D in your blood in order to get the maximum benefit from your anti-resorptive drug such as Fosamax, Actonel or Boniva.

"VITAMIN D IS INCLUDED IN MY ANTI-OSTEOPOROSIS DRUGS, SO WHY SHOULD I BE CONCERNED ABOUT VITAMIN D DEFICIENCY?"

Anti-osteoporosis drugs are now available with added vitamin D. However, a big problem is this: The vitamin D present in anti-resorptive drugs is usually 400 I.U. per day. The same quantity of vitamin D is present in "calcium preparations with D." On the bottle, it indicates that vitamin D 400 I.U. per day meets 100% of your daily requirements for vitamin D. So you assume you're taking the right amount of vitamin D. However, the fact is that most people on this dose are actually low in vitamin D and require a much larger dose as is obvious from the case studies included in this book.

IS THERE ANY DRUG THAT INCREASES BONE FORMATION?

There is a relatively new drug called Forteo (teriparatide) that acts by increasing bone formation. However, there are some concerns you have to keep in mind. Forteo has to be given by daily injection, is very costly and it may cause bone cancer.

Side-effects of Anti-Osteoporosis drugs ━━━━━━━━

Like any other drug, anti-osteoporosis drugs can cause a number of side-effects which you should be aware of. Here is a list of common as well as rare potential side-effects from these drugs.

SIDE-EFFECTS OF ANTI-OSTEOPOROSIS DRUGS.

Drug	Potential side-effects
Fosamax (alendronate) Actonel (risedronate) Boniva (Ibandronate) *All three of these drugs belong to the same family which is called Bisphosphonates.	Rare but most serious side-effect is "melting away of jaw bones" medically known as osteonecrosis. Recently, patients on these drugs were found to have increased incidence of cancer of the esophagus. Common side-effects are nausea, heartburn and stomach upset.
Evista	Serious side-effect can be cancer of the uterus. A common side-effect is hot flashes.
Estrogen Replacement Therapy	Increased risk for breast cancer, clot formation, heart attack and stroke. These risks substantially increase with prolonged use (for more than a couple of years) and especially in women older than 60 years of age.
Miacalcin	Nasal stuffiness and congestion. Rare risk for nasal bleeding.
Forteo (Teriparatide)	Rare risk for bone cancer. More common side-effect is a high calcium level in the blood.

In comparison to these anti-osteoporosis drugs, vitamin D in high doses is extremely safe and cheap. Vitamin D toxicity is extremely rare (see Chapter 24 on Vitamin D Toxicity).

Vitamin D as an Anti-Osteoporosis agent ━━━━━━━

Vitamin D plays a pivotal role in bone formation. Vitamin D exerts a direct effect on the osteoblasts, cells that lay down new bone. In addition, vitamin D in adequate amounts is essential in the proper absorption of calcium and phosphorus from your intestines. Therefore, vitamin D, calcium and phosphorus in adequate amounts are an important factor for proper bone formation to take place.

People with chronic vitamin D deficiency often end up with a serious disease called secondary hyperparathyroidism (see Chapter 6 for details). In this condition, parathyroid glands in your body start to produce a large amount of Parathyroid Hormone (PTH). This PTH excess causes an increase in bone resorption, which leads to a decrease in bone mineral density. Because vitamin D deficiency is a very common disorder, it stands to reason that secondary hyperparathyroidism is also pretty common, although it often remains undiagnosed primarily because physicians don't order a PTH blood level.

In summary, vitamin D, calcium and phosphorus in the right amounts are essential for bone formation. You can prevent osteoporosis in the first place, if you take the proper amount of vitamin D in your younger years. Even when you are diagnosed with osteopenia or osteoporosis, you can make a big difference in your bone health by taking a good dose of vitamin D.

My approach to the Treatment of Osteopenia/Osteoporosis ━━━━

When I see a patient with osteopenia or osteoporosis, first of all I investigate various causes of osteoporosis such as menopause in women, low testosterone level in men, too much thyroid hormone, steroid use etc. In addition, I always check her/his vitamin D level, which often turns out to be low. I put these patients on a good dose of vitamin D which is usually in a range of 2000-6000 units of vitamin D3 per day. Details for determining the proper dose of vitamin D are discussed in Chapter 23, Treatment of Vitamin D Deficiency.

In my patients, I monitor bone mineral density every one to two years. If a patient has a good vitamin D level, yet continues to have low bone density as estimated by the T-score on a bone DXA test, then I add an anti-osteoporosis drug. However, before I add any anti-osteoporosis drug, I discuss efficacy and potential side-effects of each of these medications and let my patient decide which potential side-effects they are willing to gamble on. In this way, my patients make an educated, well-informed decision when they choose to take an anti-osteoporosis drug.

References:

1. Bischoff-Ferrari HA, Kiel DP, et al. Dietary calcium intake and serum 25-hydroxyvitamin D status in relation to BMD among U.S. adults. *J Bone Miner Res.* 2009; 24(5):935-942.
2. De Cock C, Bruyere O, et al. Vitamin D inadequacy in French osteoporotic and osteopenic women. *Joint Bone Spine.* 2008;75(5):567-572.
3. Steele B, Serota A, et al. Vitamin D deficiency: A common occurrence in both high and low-energy fractures. *HSS J.* 2008;4(2):143-148.
4. Bruyere O, Reginster JY. Vitamin D status and response to antiosteoporotic therapy. *Womens Health* (Lond Engl). 2008;4(5):445-447.

CHAPTER 8

Vitamin D Deficiency and Steroid Use

Physicians often prescribe oral steroids to treat a number of chronic diseases such as asthma, arthritis and ulcerative colitis, to name just a few. Many patients receive epidural shots of steroids for chronic low back pain.

Most people, including many physicians, don't realize the devastating effects of steroids on vitamin D level in the body. Steroids pretty much eat away your vitamin D. Most people are low in vitamin D to start with. Steroid use further lowers their vitamin D level. These patients then suffer the consequences of vitamin D deficiency and develop severe muscle weakness and osteoporosis.

In addition, steroids directly affect the muscles and bones, worsening muscle weakness and osteoporosis. Muscle weakness primarily affects the muscles around the hips and thighs, causing difficulty in standing and walking. Consequently, these patients can easily fall. With their bones already weakened due to steroid induced osteoporosis, they easily break their hip or vertebra in the back. A hip fracture further impairs mobility and a fracture of the vertebra causes incapacitating back pain.

No drug available today effectively treats steroid-induced

osteoporosis. Here is one situation where prevention is your best treatment. Your best defense is a good dose of vitamin D. Unfortunately, many physicians don't check vitamin D level, but immediately prescribe an anti-osteoporosis drug such as alendronate (Fosamax), risedronate (Actonel) or ibandronate (Boniva) which doesn't work effectively in steroid-induced osteoporosis.

Beware! Next time some one puts you on a steroid, you must increase your daily dose of vitamin D. You'll save your bones and avoid a lot of misery in the years to come.

For more information on my strategy for treating vitamin D deficiency for those taking steroids, please see Chapter 23, Treatment of Vitamin D Deficiency.

CHAPTER 9

Vitamin D Deficiency and Immune System Diseases

What is the Immune System and what is its function? Metaphorically speaking, the Immune System is the "police" of the body. The function of the Immune System is to recognize and eliminate any bad elements such as viruses or bacteria, which can cause damage to the body.

The Immune System consists of a variety of cells with each category of cells having a unique function assigned to it. For example, some cells are specialized to fight off acute infections such as the common cold, flu and pneumonia while another type of cell deals with chronic infections such as valley fever, AIDS and tuberculosis.

Some cells are specialized to kill cancer cells. Think of cancer cells as renegade cells which have acquired special albeit abnormal characteristics. These cancer cells feed their own kind by fast replication, meanwhile starving and damaging the rest of the body by depleting the body's resources. A healthy Immune System recognizes the dangers of cancer cells and moves to destroy them.

Perhaps now you understand what an important role your

immune system plays in keeping you healthy. If you have a weak immune system, you're at risk for all sorts of infections as well as cancers.

Sometimes the Immune System itself goes haywire, seemingly becoming paranoid and mounting pre-emptive strikes against normal cells of the body, reacting as if they were dangerous and needed elimination. This is the basis of "autoimmune disorders."

For example, if your Immune System kills off your insulin producing cells (beta cells) in your pancreas, you develop Type 1 diabetes; If the target of the attack is your respiratory system, you develop asthma; If the target is nervous tissue, you develop Multiple Sclerosis (MS); If the target is the thyroid gland, you develop either Hashimoto's thyroiditis or Graves' disease; If the target is the intestines, you develop Crohn's disease or Ulcerative colitis; If the target is joints, you develop Rheumatoid arthritis or Systemic Lupus Erythematosus (SLE). Perhaps, now you can appreciate how important it is to keep your Immune System normal in order to enjoy true health!

Modern research has clearly established that vitamin D plays a vital role in the normal functioning of the Immune System. This is a breakthrough discovery! So far, traditional medicine has ignored the Immune System side of the equation to fight off infections and cancers because it could not offer any substantial remedy. For infections, all it could offer was antibiotics. For cancers, all it could offer was chemotherapy, radiation and surgery. For autoimmune disorders, all it could offer was to suppress the abnormal overactive immune system. There was no effective way to boost up your own immunity to fight off infections or a way to normalize the abnormal immune system. However, vitamin D as an immune system modulator can change it all!

Common Colds, Flu, *Swine Flu*

Vitamin D builds up the Immune System to fight off viruses that cause the common cold and influenza (Flu). Studies have shown that individuals low in vitamin D are at increased risk for common colds. In a study (1) recently published in the Archives of Internal Medicine, researchers found a clear link between vitamin D deficiency and common colds.

Can vitamin D supplement prevent *Swine Flu?*

From the outbreak of *Swine Flu* in the summer of 2009, there are several anecdotal reports from physicians who noted the occurence of *Swine Flu* was rare in people taking vitamin D supplements compared to those who did not. In my own clinical practice, only one patient had *Swine Flu* in the Fall of 2009 despite the fact that *Swine Flu* was widespread in our community.

Asthma

There is strong link between vitamin D deficiency and asthma. In the U.S., the prevalence of asthma has increased dramatically from about 3 % in the 1970's to about 8% in recent years. New England tops the nation in the prevalence of asthma. In this region during winter, there is inadequate UVB from the sun for the synthesis of vitamin D. Therefore, scientists wondered whether vitamin D deficiency could be responsible for the development of asthma and whether vitamin D supplementation could be helpful in the prevention and treatment of asthma.

Sound medical research has shown that vitamin D plays a significant role in the development of the Immune System and lungs during fetal growth. Studies have shown that vitamin D supplementation during pregnancy can substantially reduce the risk of asthma in a child (2). Experts in the field of asthma speculate the epidemic of asthma to be linked to the epidemic of vitamin D deficiency, as both of these epidemics started in the last few decades. Children and adults low in vitamin D are at an increased risk for upper respiratory tract infections which often trigger wheezing and asthma attacks in susceptible individuals.

Severe asthma is treated with steroids, but sometimes patients are resistant to steroids. This is known as steroid-resistant asthma. Vitamin D has been shown to make steroid treatment more effective in these individuals.

Tuberculosis

Patients with tuberculosis are particularly low in vitamin D. Typically, tuberculosis affects individuals who are poor and live in crowded dwellings in inner cities coated with pollution. Poverty leads to malnutrition and lack of sun exposure leads to vitamin D deficiency. In particular, children living under these socioeconomic conditions often become victims of tuberculosis.

In one study (3) at a tuberculosis clinic in the U.K., researchers found that vitamin D was low in all but one child. In other studies, researchers have found vitamin D supplements to be a helpful adjunct in the treatment of tuberculosis, especially in those cases resistant to the usual drug treatment.

Rheumatoid Arthritis, Systemic Lupus Erythematosus (SLE) and Other Rheumatologic Diseases

Vitamin D deficiency is extremely common in patients with autoimmune disorders such as rheumatoid arthritis, lupus (SLE) and various other rheumatologic diseases. This is an area of intense research. Mounting scientific evidence links low vitamin D to development of rheumatoid arthritis and lupus.

At a meeting in 2008 of the European Union League Against

Rheumatism, Irish researchers reported that 70% of patients at their rheumatology clinic had vitamin D deficiency. To define vitamin D deficiency, they used a level of vitamin D less than 21ng/ml. If they had used 30 ng/ml. as a cutoff level for low vitamin D, a level that most experts agree upon, the number of patients with low vitamin D would have been even higher, perhaps close to 90%.

Several studies link a low level of vitamin D to rheumatoid arthritis. An excellent study published in 2004 showed that vitamin D intake was inversely associated with risk of rheumatoid arthritis. People with a higher intake of vitamin D were at low risk for the development of rheumatoid arthritis (4).

Several studies also indicate low vitamin D playing a role in patients with SLE (Systemic Lupus Erythematosus). In one study, researchers from Canada found that over 50% of their SLE patients were very low in vitamin D (5). In another study, researchers found 67% of their SLE patients to be vitamin D deficient and there was a trend for all patients to be low in vitamin D (6).

In my experience, most patients with rheumatologic diseases such as rheumatoid arthritis, fibromyalgia and chronic body aches and pains are low in vitamin D. With proper supplementation with vitamin D, they see a dramatic improvement in their symptoms.

Multiple Sclerosis (M.S.) ━━━━━━━━━━━━━━━━━

Multiple sclerosis is a chronic debilitating disease that affects the brain, spinal cord and the nerves. It usually starts in young adulthood and practically robs a person's quality of life. There are recurring episodes of neurologic dysfunction which can result in partial or complete loss of function of an organ. Usual symptoms are loss of vision, difficulty in speech, lack of balance, tremors, loss of bladder control, vomiting, and sometimes paralysis of an arm or leg.

While the exact cause of M.S. remains unknown, genetics, geographic location and immune dysfunction play a significant role in causing and perpetuating M.S.; Researchers have known for a long time that M.S. is primarily is a disease of northern Europe, the northern U.S. and Canada. It is rare in Africa and Asia. Even in the U.S., its prevalence in the south is 50% less than in the north.

In order to find the exact cause of M.S., most researchers have focused on finding an environmental factor, such as a virus. However, all that research has failed miserably.

Some researchers, on the other hand, looked at the obvious: M.S. occurs more frequently in northern areas with less sunshine. They speculated on the role of vitamin D deficiency in causing M.S. This quest finally led to the landmark experimental studies (7, 8) in which vitamin D (as 1,25 vitamin D3) supplementation completely prevented M.S. in animal models. Vitamin D therapy also prevented the progression of M.S. in these experimental animals. These miraculous findings led researchers to believe that vitamin D is a natural inhibitor of M.S.

Based on these findings, researchers in the field of M.S. now recommend that vitamin D supplementation be an integral part of treatment of individuals with M.S. In addition, those who are genetically at a high risk for developing M.S. should be supplemented with vitamin D.

Unfortunately, in real life, many experts treating patients with M.S. pay little if any attention to vitamin D level. They simply stay focused on drug therapy. Most patients receive steroids, which further lowers vitamin D in those who are already low in vitamin D to begin with.

In addition to steroids, there are other, relatively new drugs to treat M.S.; These drugs are quite expensive. They do give some relief of symptoms, but at the expense of severely suppressing the immune system, which makes you prone to serious, life-threatening infections. In addition, these drugs have other horrendous side-effects such as risk for lymphoma.

Vitamin D, which is cheap and virtually without any side-effects, is completely ignored. I am not against M.S. drugs. They have their place, but physicians should also pay close attention to vitamin D deficiency and treat it aggressively.

I sometimes encounter patients with M.S. who come to see me for medical problems other than M.S.; These patients are under the care of experts for the treatment of M.S.; In each one of these M.S. patients, their vitamin D level was quite low when I checked it. None of them were educated by their M.S. experts about the link between low vitamin D and M.S. I find it rather distressing. Again, another reason to write this book!

CASE STUDY

Anna consulted me primarily for her thyroid problem. As it turned out, she also suffered from M.S. for 13 years and had been under the care of M.S. specialists. Over the years, her M.S. had gradually worsened. Currently, she was on steroids and interferon therapy. Her M.S. specialists advised her to add more drugs as her M.S. was not under control.

When I told her about the link between vitamin D and M.S., she was truly amazed. No other physician had ever mentioned it to her. I placed her on vitamin D3 at 2000 I.U. a day and gradually increased it to 8000 I.U. a day while monitoring her vitamin D and calcium level in the blood.

Ten months later, she had her yearly follow-up MRI scan which showed that her M.S. disease had actually improved. Anna was thrilled and so was I!

Vitamin D supplementation should be an important part of

treating patients with M.S. In these patients, a good level of vitamin D (a level between 50-100 ng/ml or 125-250 nmol/L) should be targeted. How to achieve this level is discussed in Chapter 23, Treatment of Vitamin D Deficiency.

Autoimmune Diabetes Mellitus (Type 1 Diabetes) ━━━━━━

Type 1 diabetes mellitus (DM Type 1) usually affects younger individuals, often children. Rarely, it can affect older persons.

DM Type 1 is an autoimmune disease. In simple terms, your immune system starts malfunctioning. It misidentifies your own insulin producing cells in the pancreas as foreign and starts destroying them. It mounts an ongoing attack on your insulin producing cells until it eventually kills them all. Consequently, you can't produce any more insulin, your blood glucose escalates and you're diagnosed with diabetes.

VITAMIN D LEVEL IN TYPE 1 DM PATIENTS

I test vitamin D level in all of my patients with DM Type 1. I find it to be low in virtually all of them. My experience is in line with other researchers in this field. In a recently published study in the *Journal of Pediatrics*, researchers from the Joslin Diabetes Center noted that the vast majority of their Type 1 diabetic patients were low in vitamin D (9). The study was done in children and teenagers.

CAN VITAMIN D DEFICIENCY CAUSE TYPE 1 DIABETES MELLITUS? CAN IT BE PREVENTED WITH VITAMIN D SUPPLEMENTATION?

True researchers (the ones NOT working for drug companies) were intrigued with the possibility that vitamin D deficiency could be causing DM Type 1 by interfering with the normal functioning of the immune system. Indeed, this turns out to be the case. Ground breaking research from Finland showed a clear relationship between vitamin D deficiency and risk for developing Type 1 diabetes. It also showed Type 1 diabetes can be prevented by adequate vitamin D supplementation (10).

This study (10) began in 1966 when a total of 10,821 children born in 1966 in northern Finland were enrolled in the study. Frequency of vitamin D supplementation was recorded during the first year of life. At that time, the recommended dose of vitamin D for infants in Finland was 2000 I.U. per day. These children were then followed for 31 years for the development of Type 1 diabetes. Researchers made the amazing discovery that those children who received the daily recommended dose of 2000 I.U. of vitamin D during the first year of their life, had an almost 80% reduction in the risk for the development of Type 1 diabetes compared to those children who received less vitamin D.

This is an astounding study! If some drug achieved this kind of results, it would hit the headlines and become the standard of care at once. Sadly, even many diabetes experts are not aware of this great study.

Investigators in the U.S. continue to spend millions of dollars in their pursuit of a "drug" to prevent Type 1 diabetes. So far, this kind of research has produced disappointing results. Amazingly, they have largely ignored the strong evidence that shows the outstanding role of vitamin D in preventing Type 1 diabetes. Vitamin D is not a drug. There is no glory or huge profits in simply telling people to take enough vitamin D.

It is interesting to note that the recommended allowance of vitamin D for infants in Finland was reduced from 2000 I.U. to 1000 I.U. per day in 1975 and then further reduced to 400 I.U. per day in 1992. (For comparison, in the U.S. it has been 200 I.U. a day). This reduction in the daily allowance had no scientific basis except the observation that this amount of vitamin D is present in a teaspoonful of cod-liver oil which has long been considered safe and effective in preventing rickets.

In the last decades, the incidence of Type 1 diabetes in Finland has been climbing which is most likely related to the decrease in the daily recommended allowance of vitamin D. As of 1999, Finland has the highest reported incidence of Type 1 diabetes in the world (11). In Finland, the yearly sunshine and therefore vitamin D skin synthesis is much lower compared to more southern areas. Therefore, the population in Finland is at even higher risk for vitamin D deficiency.

In another excellent study (12), researchers found vitamin D supplementation during infancy can significantly reduce the risk for developing Type 1 diabetes. This study was carried out in seven centers in different countries across a variety of populations in Europe.

Autoimmune Thyroid Diseases ▬▬▬▬▬▬▬▬▬▬▬▬

Autoimmune thyroid disease has a wide range of manifestations: It is the most common cause of underactive thyroid (technically known as hypothyroidism). In some individuals, it can cause overactive thyroid (technically known as hyperthyroidism). When autoimmune thyroid disease causes underactive thyroid, it is called **Hashimoto's thyroiditis** and when it causes overactive thyroid, it is called **Graves' disease**.

The usual symptoms of underactive thyroid are fatigue, weight gain, mood disorders, dizziness, muscle cramps, cold intolerance, hair loss, frequent menses and memory loss.

The usual symptoms of overactive thyroid are: irritability, hyperactivity, heart palpitations, tremors, shakiness, excessive sweating, heat intolerance, weight loss, bulging eyes, infrequent menses, osteoporosis, anxiety and panic attacks. Rarely, patients can develop psychotic symptoms such as hallucinations, delusions and irrational behavior. Sometimes patients can have predominant eye symptoms such as watery bulging eyes and double vision. Very rarely, patients can also have excessive thickening and swelling of their skin in the lower legs.

If hypothyroidism remains untreated for a long period of time, a person can lapse into a coma and death can occur.

Typically, physicians treat underactive thyroid by giving thyroid hormone in the form of a pill. In the case of overactive thyroid due to Graves' disease, we either give an anti-thyroid drug or destroy the thyroid gland by exposure to radioactive iodine. Almost all Graves' disease patients treated with radioactive iodine end up with underactive thyroid (hypothyroid). They then need to take a thyroid hormone pill for the rest of their life.

In medical literature, genetics is the main factor recognized as the contributory factor for causing autoimmune thyroid disease and of course, there's nothing you can do about that. However, I check vitamin D level in all of my patients with autoimmune thyroid disease and find it to be low in most of them. I suspect vitamin D to be a factor in causing autoimmune thyroid disease. Interestingly, in a recent experimental study from UCLA School of Medicine, vitamin D deficiency was found to cause Graves' disease in animals (13).

In addition, I find two other factors to be commonly present in patients with autoimmune thyroid disease. These are: fear and a high carbohydrate diet. Both of these factors are likely causative factors for autoimmune thyroid disease.

Inflammatory Bowel Disease (IBD) ━━━━━━━━━━━━

Inflammatory Bowel Disease (IBD) is a chronic disease of the intestines which not only diminishes quality of life, but often results in debilitating complications. There are two main clinical forms of

IBD: **Ulcerative colitis and Crohn's disease.**
The usual symptoms are:
- Bloody diarrhea
- Abdominal cramping
- Excessive gas
- Weight loss
- Fatigue

Complications of IBD include:
- Perforation of the intestines
- Fistula formation
- Intestinal obstruction
- Colon cancer

The medical treatment for IBD patients consists of a wide array of drugs, all of which aim to reduce inflammation of the intestines. Most patients receive steroids in high doses with their serious side-effects including reduction of vitamin D level. Many of the other drugs also have serious side-effects such as risk for tuberculosis, renal failure and lymphoma. Despite the use of these drugs, patients often continue to have relapses of symptoms. Many patients end up losing part of their intestines. Colon cancer is also much more common in patients with ulcerative colitis than in the general population.

To me, the current treatment is a band-aid approach. We physicians keep trying to suppress inflammation by one drug or another without examining the very basic question: What is the real cause for the inflammation and what can we do to treat this root cause? Based on my own clinical experience and extensive scientific studies in this field, I developed a deeper approach for treating my patients with IBD, discussed later in this chapter. First, let's investigate the relationship between IBD and low vitamin D.

THE LINK BETWEEN IBD AND VITAMIN D DEFICIENCY

Vitamin D is almost always low in patients with IBD. As we know, low vitamin D leads to malfunction of the immune system. It is intuitive to conclude that Vitamin D deficiency plays a vital role in the development and progression of IBD. Once IBD develops, patients often spend more time indoors, in hospitals and recovering at home which further lowers their vitamin D level.

In addition, the small amount of vitamin D that people get from their food is also lost in patients with IBD due to intestinal malabsorption. Consequently, vitamin D level in these patients drops even lower. Low vitamin D further impairs the immune system and thus a vicious cycle starts: low vitamin D causes IBD which causes further reduction in vitamin D which then causes further disruption of the immune system and more progression of IBD.

CAN VITAMIN D SUPPLEMENTATION HELP PATIENTS WITH IBD?

The answer is yes!

One experimental study showed that vitamin D can prevent the symptoms of experimental IBD (14). In two clinical human studies, fish oil (a rich source of vitamin D) was shown to decrease the severity of IBD (15,16).

My Approach to the Treatment of Autoimmune Diseases. ▬▬▬

I do treat the symptoms of an autoimmune disease with traditional medical practices such as giving thyroid hormone to underactive thyroid patients or giving insulin to Type 1 diabetic patients or giving steroids for ulcerative colitis flare-ups. However, I also look deeper and treat factors that resulted in the development of the autoimmune disease in the first place. If you don't treat the underlying cause of immune dysfunction, it will continue to erupt to the surface in the form of another autoimmune disease. In medical literature, it is well known that a person with one autoimmune disease is at high risk for developing other autoimmune diseases.

What causes Autoimmune Diseases? ━━━━━━━━━━━

1. **Genetics**

   Autoimmune diseases tend to congregate in families. You're at high risk for developing an autoimmune disease if you have a family history of these diseases. However, not every genetically predisposed individual (not even twins) develops an autoimmune disease. Acquired factors play an important role in bringing out the disease in these individuals with genetic predisposition. These acquired factors are discussed below.

2. **Vitamin D Deficiency**

   As I have elaborated in this chapter, there is strong evidence to incriminate low vitamin D as an important factor in the causation of autoimmune diseases.

3. **Diet**

   Extensive scientific studies have clearly established that diet plays an important role in the causation and progression of autoimmune diseases. Certain genetically predisposed individuals are not able to digest starches and sugars properly. The partially digested starches and sugars provide fertile grounds for bacteria and yeast to thrive in the intestines, causing "bacterial overgrowth." The byproducts of these micro-organisms cause inflammation of the intestinal walls, making them more permeable. Large molecules of partially digested food can then leak into the blood stream. This is called Leaky Gut Syndrome, which in turn, activates your immune system unnecessarily which then starts to malfunction. Therefore, starches and sugars play an important role in causing and perpetuating autoimmune disease.

4. **Stress**

   Stress is a well known factor in the causation of autoimmune disease. Stress, especially in the form of fear, causes your body to produce excess amounts of cortisol, a hormone produced by the adrenal glands. An excessive amount of cortisol is known to weaken the immune system.

Based upon the four factors described above, I give the following advice to my patients with autoimmune diseases:

Genetics, of course, you can't change but you can do a lot about the other three factors.

1. **Vitamin D Supplements**

   Check your vitamin D level (for details please refer to Chapter 22, Diagnosis of Vitamin D Deficiency). Aim to keep your vitamin D level between 50 and 100 ng/ml (125 nmol/L to 250 nmol/L). To achieve these levels, most people require vitamin D supplementation in large doses (See Chapter 23, Treatment of Vitamin D Deficiency).

2. **Low Carbohydrate Diet**

   Reduce starches and most carbohydrates in your diet. I tell my patients to eliminate all cereals, oatmeal, bread of any color or type, other bakery products, pasta of any type, rice of any color or type, corn, potatoes, sweet potatoes, sugar, milk, commercial fruit juices, soy, corn syrup, fructose syrup, ice cream and other desserts.

   Instead, eat poultry, meats, egg whites, vegetables, fruits (not fruit juices), yogurt, nuts and seeds.

For example, I recommend the following food items:
Breakfast:
- Eggs (egg whites only if you have cholesterol problem or have heart disease)
- Yogurt, plain. You can add fresh strawberries, blueberries or sprinkle some powdered cinnamon.
- Coffee or tea.

Lunch or Dinner:
- Garden salad
- Chicken, turkey, beef or lamb

- Vegetables
- Nuts
- Fruits

A full description of my recommended diet is out of the scope of this book. However, you can obtain my diet from my website: www. DoctorZaidi.com

This is a truly healthy diet. I recommend it to most of my patients, not only those with autoimmune diseases, but also those with Type 2 Diabetes, Pre-Diabetes, and Metabolic Syndrome.

For those with Ulcerative Colitis and Crohn's disease, I recommend a wonderful book, "Breaking the Vicious Cycle" by Elaine Gottschall. Website: www.scdiet.com

3. **Stress Management**
   A discussion about stress and its management could fill a book – literally! Keep a watch for my upcoming book, "Freedom From Stress" without the use of medications. In the meantime, here's a brief overview.

THE ORIGIN OF FEAR

What is the origin of fear? It originates when you're thinking about the future. I call it the "What If Syndrome."
- What if I miss my flight?
- What if Wall Street goes down?
- What if I lose my job?
- What if I have another attack of asthma? Crohn's disease? Heart disease?
- What if I develop diabetes and die a miserable death like my mother?

If you look at your fear closely, you'll understand its true origin.

You realize that you're holding on to some negative experience of your own or of other people (Maybe you read about it or saw it on T.V.). You do not want it to happen to you ever, because it was (or could be) so painful. The mere thought that it may happen triggers a wave of fear and anxiety in you. Fear causes a release of adrenaline and cortisol from your adrenal glands. Both of these hormones damage your body. Adrenaline raises your blood pressure, increases your heart rate and may even cause chest tightness and chest pain. Cortisol plays havoc on your immune system.

So, how can I be Free of Fear?

You can be free of fear if you use logic. Obviously "what if" or "what may' is a creation of your own mind, isn't it? It may or may not happen. It's not a problem in reality, not happening at this moment, right? Therefore, it's a phantom, an illusion. If and when it happens, at "that time, in the present moment," you'll be able to take care of it.

For example, you're stuck in traffic on your way to the airport and there's nothing you can do about it. You start worrying. "What if I miss my flight and then I'll miss my interview for this job I really want and my best chance to get this dream job will evaporate" and on and on. You get so fearful from the drama that your mind creates that you may end up having chest tightness and pain and find yourself heading to a hospital. **Or** you can choose not to think about 'what if,' but instead stay in the present moment, focus on your driving and arrive at the airport safely. You may or may not be late. If you are late, you will deal with it. Therefore, live in the Now, stay in reality and you won't have any fear.

Take action in the present moment. For example, eat right, exercise regularly and take vitamin D every day. There's a good chance you won't develop diabetes. However, if you just keep worrying about diabetes and don't take any actions, you may develop diabetes. Take real actions in the present moment and don't worry about the results.

REFERENCES:

1. Ginde A, Mansbach J, et al. Association between serum 25-hydroxy vitamin D level and upper respiratory tract infection in the third National Health and Nutrition Examination Survey. Arch Int Med 2009;169(4):384-390.

2. Litonjua AA, Weiss ST. Is vitamin D deficiency to blame for the asthma epidemic. J Allergy Clin Immunol. 2007;120(5):1031-1035.

3. Williams B, Williams AJ, Anderson ST. Vitamin D deficiency and insufficiency in children with tuberculosis. Pediatr Infect Dis J. 2008;27(10):941-942.

4. Merlino LA, Curtis J, Mikuls TR et al. Vitamin D intake is inversely associated with rheumatoid arthritis: results from the Iowa Women's Health Study. Arthritis Rheum 2004;50:72-77.

5. Huisman AM, White KP, Algra A, et al. Vitamin D levels in women with systemic lupus erythematosus and fibromyalgia. J Rheumatol 2001;28:2535-2539.

6. Kamen DL, Cooper GS, Bouali H, et al. Vitamin D deficiency in systemic lupus erythematosus. Autoimmune Rev 2006;5:114-117.

7. Hayes CE. Vitamin D. a natural inhibitor of multiple sclerosis. Proc Nutr Soc. 2000;59(4):531-535.

8. Raghuwanshi A, Joshi SS, Christakos S. Vitamin D and multiple sclerosis. J Cell Biochem.2008;105(2):338-343.

9. Svoren BM, Volkening LK, Wood JR, Laffel LM. Significant vitamin D deficiency in youth with Type 1 diabetes mellitus. J Pediatr.2009;154(1):132-134.

10. Hypponen E, Laara E, Reunanen A, et al. Intake of vitamin D and risk of Type 1 diabetes: a birth-cohort study. Lancet 2001;358:1500-1503.

11. Onkamo P, Vaananen S, Karvonen M, Tuomilchto J. Worldwide increase in incidence of Type 1 diabetes: the analysis of the data on published incidence trends. Diabetologia 1999;42:1395-1403.
12. The EURODIAB Substudy 2 Study Group. Vitamin D supplementation in early childhood and risk for Type 1 (insulin- dependent) diabetes mellitus. Diabetologia 1999;42:51-54.
13. Misharin A, Hewison M et al. Vitamin D deficiency modulates Graves' hyperthyroidism induced in BALB/c mice by thyrotropin receptor immunization. Endocrinology. 2009, 150(2):1051-1060.
14. Cantorna MT, Munsick C et al. 1,25-Dihydroxycholecalciferol prevents and ameliorates symptoms of experimental murine inflammatory bowel disease. J Nutr 2000;130:2648-2652.
15. Aslan A, Triadafilopoulos G. Fish oil fatty acid supplementation in active ulcerative colitis: a double-blind, placebo-controlled crossover study. Am J Gastroenterol 1992; 87:432-437.
16. Stenson WF, Cort D et al. Dietary supplementation with fish oil in ulcerative colitis. Ann Intern Med 1992;116:609-614.

CHAPTER 10

Vitamin D Deficiency and Cancer

Dermatologists have successfully hammered one thought into all of us: sun exposure may cause skin cancer, so wear sunscreen while you're out in the sun. What dermatologists don't tell us is that the vitamin D we get from sunshine can also prevent serious cancers such as breast, colon, pancreatic and prostate cancers.

Mounting scientific evidence shows a strong link between vitamin D deficiency and cancer. Wouldn't it be wonderful if we could prevent cancer by optimizing vitamin D level in the body? Even in patients with a diagnosis of cancer, proper vitamin D supplementation plays an important role in treating cancer and preventing its recurrence.

What promotes cancer growth?

In the last two decades, research has clearly shown two factors can promote growth of cancer: **Vitamin D deficiency and Insulin Resistance Syndrome**.

First, let's examine how cancer develops. In your body, old cells are constantly dying and fresh new cells are being born. In other words, there is a continuing cycle of death and birth of cells. There is also a fine balance between the death and the birth of cells.

Vitamin D is involved in the death of cells and insulin is involved in the growth of new cells. Now consider a scenario where vitamin D is low in the body and insulin level is high. Both of these factors cause a shift in the normal balance of the death and birth of cells. Low vitamin D causes a decrease in the death of cells and a high insulin level causes an increase in the growth of cells. The net result is an enormous increase in the number of cells. This is exactly what happens when you have cancer; an unlimited growth of *abnormal* cells in your body.

A high level of insulin is present in people with Insulin Resistance Syndrome (also known as Metabolic Syndrome). Briefly, Insulin Resistance Syndrome consists of obesity, hypertension, low HDL cholesterol, high triglycerides, pre-diabetes or diabetes, polycystic ovary syndrome and high uric acid level. You don't have to have all of these features. Just a couple of them are enough to have a diagnosis of Insulin Resistance Syndrome. Some complications of Insulin Resistance Syndrome include: coronary artery disease, stroke and fatty liver. For an in depth look at Insulin Resistance Syndrome, please read my book, "Take Charge of Your Diabetes."

We could call vitamin D deficiency and high insulin level two important promoters of cancer. It's interesting to note that vitamin D deficiency has been shown to worsen Insulin Resistance Syndrome which results in a further increase in insulin level.

In addition, obesity, which often plays a central role in Insulin Resistance Syndrome, also causes vitamin D deficiency. Obesity is the obvious common denominator for insulin resistance and vitamin D deficiency. For a long time, physicians have known obesity to be a strong risk factor for cancer. Now we understand that vitamin D deficiency and insulin resistance are two pathways for how obesity is linked to cancer.

Both vitamin D deficiency and Insulin Resistance Syndrome have reached epidemic proportions, affecting hundreds of millions of people around the world. What's alarming is that both vitamin D deficiency and Insulin Resistance Syndrome are getting worse. It is intuitive to predict that we will continue to see increasingly large numbers of cancer cases as time passes.

Evidence for the Link Between Vitamin D Deficiency and Cancer ▬

Is there is any evidence to show a link between low vitamin D level and cancer? The answer is yes. The evidence is overwhelming! A large number of studies have shown a link between low vitamin D and cancer. Researchers from the University of California-San Diego published an excellent article (1) in the *American Journal of Public Health* in 2006. They analyzed scientific studies investigating the relationship between vitamin D level and cancer risk. These researchers found 30 studies on colon cancer, 13 studies on breast cancer, 26 studies on prostate cancer and 7 studies on ovarian cancer. In the majority of these studies, researchers concluded that people with a good level of vitamin D had a lower risk for developing these cancers.

Scientific studies have also found higher rates of cancer mortality in regions with a higher latitude (less vitamin D from sunshine) as compared to regions closer to the equator (more vitamin D from sunshine).

Physicians have made another interesting observation: people diagnosed with cancer in the months of summer and autumn have better survival rates as compared to individuals diagnosed with the same type of cancer in the months of winter. The logical explanation for this difference in survival is that there is more vitamin D from sunshine in the months of summer and autumn as compared to the months of winter.

Therefore, vitamin D level at the time of diagnosis of cancer can have a prognostic value. In one such study, researchers from

Norway followed 123 patients with prostate cancer and found that patients with a good level of vitamin D at the time of diagnosis of prostate cancer had a better survival rate (2).

Can Vitamin D help in the treatment of cancer?

The answer is yes!

Vitamin D not only helps to prevent cancer, but it also helps in the treatment of cancer. A researcher from Harvard Medical School published an excellent article (3) in 2005 citing the enormous evidence which strongly supports the anti-cancer role of vitamin D supplementation in patients with colon cancer.

In the case of breast cancer, the role of vitamin D as an anticancer agent is promising. In the case of prostate cancer, it appears that the more active form of vitamin D, known as 1,25, $(OH)_2$ vitamin D, provides anti-cancer activity.

Amazingly, many oncologists don't seriously consider the great anti-cancer benefits of vitamin D. Some oncologists who stay updated on current knowledge may casually recommend vitamin D to their patients.

What I've seen in my patients is usually something like this: If a patient brings up the subject of vitamin D, the oncologist might say, "Yeah, it's a good idea. You should take vitamin D." Unfortunately, that's often the end of the advice. Vitamin D level is not checked. Dosage amount is not discussed. The patient usually ends up taking vitamin D on their own at dose of 400 I.U. per day, which according to the bottle label, meets 100% of the daily recommended dose. When these patients come to see me for some other reason, such as diabetes, I check their vitamin D level. In most cases, their vitamin D level is low, despite being on the recommended dose of 400 I.U. per day.

So beware and take charge of your vitamin D status and

supplementation! In Chapters 22 and 23 on Diagnosis and Treatment of Vitamin D Deficiency, you can educate yourself on how to take charge of your vitamin D needs.

CASE STUDY

Martin, a Caucasian male, was diagnosed with colon cancer at the age of 49. The cancer was quite aggressive and had spread to his liver at the time of diagnosis. The prognosis for Martin was poor. No one in his family had colon cancer. "Why did it happen to me? I'm not that old." Martin said.

I evaluated him for vitamin D deficiency and Insulin Resistance Syndrome. Martin had both of these conditions. His vitamin D level was 20 ng/ml., which is quite low. He also had abdominal obesity, low HDL cholesterol, high triglycerides, high insulin level and an abnormal glucose tolerance test. Based on these findings, I diagnosed him with Insulin Resistance Syndrome.

While his oncologist treated Martin with chemotherapy, I treated his Insulin Resistance Syndrome and Vitamin D Deficiency. Together, we have achieved amazing results. Three years later, Martin continues to be cancer-free.

REFERENCES:

1. Garland CF, Garland FC, Gorham ED et al. The role of vitamin D in cancer prevention. *Am J Pub Health.* 2006;96(2):252-26.
2. Tretli S, Hernes E, Berg JP, et al. Association Between serum 25(OH)D and death from prostate cancer. *Br J Cancer.* 2009;100(3):450-454.
3. Giovannucci E. The epidemiology of vitamin D and cancer incidence and mortality: a review(United States). *Cancer Causes Control.* 2005;16(2):83-95.

CHAPTER 11

Vitamin D Deficiency and Heart Disease

When it comes to heart disease, everyone thinks of cholesterol. What most people don't know is that vitamin D deficiency is also linked to heart disease. Is there any scientific evidence to show the relationship between vitamin D deficiency and heart disease?

Evidence for the Link Between Vitamin D Deficiency and Heart Disease.

Scientific evidence to show the link between vitamin D deficiency and heart disease continues to grow. In an article (1) published in 1989 in *Lancet*, a respected British Medical Journal, a researcher noted a relationship between latitude and heart disease: the farther you live from the equator, the lower you are in vitamin D and the higher your risk for heart disease.

Over the years, numerous studies continue to show a relationship between low vitamin D level and heart disease. However, this vital information hardly received any public attention until 2008 when two studies finally got the attention of the news media.

In the first study (2), published in January 2008 in *Circulation* (the official journal of the American Heart Association), researchers followed 1739 participants for the development of heart disease. The mean follow-up was 5.4 years. These researchers found a 2-fold increase in the risk for heart disease in individuals who had a low level of vitamin D.

In the second study (3), published in the June 9, 2008 issue of the *Archives of Internal Medicine* (the official journal of the American Medical Association), investigators looked at the level of vitamin D in men who developed a heart attack during a 10 year follow-up period. The results were stunning: the lower the vitamin D level, the higher the risk for heart attack. Men whose vitamin D level was at least 30 ng/ml had half the risk of a heart attack compared to men who had a vitamin D level below 30 ng/ml.

How Vitamin D may Prevent Heart Disease. ━━━━━━━

A recent provocative study (4) looked into the precise mechanism for how vitamin D may prevent coronary heart disease. The researchers found that vitamin D was able to prevent the uptake of LDL cholesterol by the cells in the arterial walls, which is the main reason for narrowing of the coronary arteries. In addition, vitamin D has been shown to decrease insulin resistance and blood vessel inflammation, two other important factors that cause coronary heart disease.

Take Vitamin D Supplements To Prevent Heart Disease ━━━━━

In the last three decades, heart disease has become so prevalent that it's the number one killer in the U.S.; During the same time period, vitamin D deficiency has grown to epidemic proportions. Compelling scientific evidence indicates that vitamin D appears to be a significant factor in heart disease. Vitamin D is cheap, has virtual no side-effects and has many benefits in addition to cardiovascular benefits. Isn't it time to get on board and take charge of your vitamin D needs?

In addition to diet and exercise, you should consider taking vitamin D supplements in order to prevent heart disease. For details on vitamin D supplements, please refer to Chapter 23, Treatment of Vitamin D Deficiency.

REFERENCES:

1. Fleck A. Latitude and ischemic heart disease. *Lancet.* 1989;1:613.
2. Wang TJ, Pencina MJ, Booth SL, et al. Vitamin D deficiency and risk of cardiovascular disease. *Circulation.*2008;117:503-511.
3. Giovannucci E, Liu Y, Hollis BW, Rimm EB. 25-hydroxyvitamin D and risk of myocardial infarction in men. A prospective study. *Arch Intern Med.* 2008;168:1174-1180.
4. Oh J, Weng S, Felton SK et al.1,25(OH)$_2$ vitamin d inhibits foam cell formation and suppresses macrophage cholesterol uptake in patients with type 2 diabetes mellitus. *Circulation.*2009;120:687-698.

CHAPTER 12

Vitamin D Deficiency and Diabetes Mellitus

Diabetes has reached epidemic proportions in the U.S. and around the globe. There are two types of diabetes mellitus: Type 1, which affects about 5% of diabetics and Type 2 which affects about 95% of diabetics.

TYPE 1 DIABETES

Type 1 diabetes typically affects children and young adults. Rarely, it can develop in older individuals as well.

The usual symptoms of Type 1 Diabetes are:
- Excessive, frequent urination
- Excessive thirst
- Blurry vision
- Weight loss
- Fatigue

A less frequent but potentially life-threatening presentation of diabetes is known as DKA (Diabetic Keto Acidosis). In this condition, you develop shortness of breath, nausea or vomiting, abdominal pain, dehydration, dizziness, fatigue, somnolence, disorientation and even coma. Death can occur if this condition is not promptly treated.

Insulin is the treatment for patients with DM Type 1. Treatment is necessary for the rest of your life.

The Relationship Between Vitamin D Deficiency and Type 1 Diabetes ▪

Type 1 diabetes develops due to malfunctioning of the immune system. As I discussed in Chapter 9, mounting scientific evidence indicates that vitamin D plays a vital role in the normal functioning of the immune system and vitamin D deficiency can lead to the malfunctioning of the immune system. Consequently, your own immune system starts to attack and kill your own insulin producing cells in the pancreas. Once you are *unable* to produce insulin, you develop Type 1 diabetes.

Evidence for the Link Between Vitamin D Deficiency and Type 1 Diabetes ─────

Researchers have investigated the level of vitamin D in patients with Type 1 diabetes and found it to be low in the vast majority of these patients. In a recently published study in *the Journal of Pediatrics*, researchers from the Joslin Diabetes Center noted that the vast majority of their Type 1 diabetic patients were low in vitamin D (1). The study was done in children and teenagers.

In my clinical practice, I check vitamin D level in all of my Type 1 diabetic patients and find it to be low in virtually all of them.

Evidence that Vitamin D can Prevent Type 1 Diabetes ──────

As I discussed in Chapter 9, scientific evidence now exists to show that proper vitamin D supplementation can prevent Type 1 diabetes.

One such study comes from Finland. This study (2) began in 1966 when a total of 10,821 children born in 1966 in northern Finland were enrolled in the study. Frequency of vitamin D supplementation was recorded during the first year of life. At that time, the recommended dose of vitamin D for infants in Finland was 2000 I.U. per day. These children were then followed for 31 years for the development of Type 1 diabetes. Researchers made the amazing discovery that those children who received the daily recommended dose of 2000 I.U. of Vitamin D during the first year of their life, had an almost 80% reduction in the risk for the development of Type 1 diabetes compared to those children who received less vitamin D.

This is a ground breaking study! If some drug achieved this kind of results, it would hit the headlines and become the standard of care at once. Sadly, even many diabetes experts are not aware of this astounding study even though the study was published in 2001 in the prestigious British medical journal called *Lancet*.

Investigators in the U.S. continue to spend millions of dollars in their pursuit of a "drug" to prevent Type 1 diabetes. So far, this kind of research has produced disappointing results. Amazingly, they have largely ignored the strong evidence that shows the outstanding role of vitamin D in preventing Type 1 diabetes. Vitamin D is not a drug. There is no glory or huge profits in simply telling people to take enough vitamin D.

It is interesting to note that the recommended allowance of vitamin D for infants in Finland was reduced from 2000 I.U. to 1000 I.U. per day in 1975 and then further reduced to 400 I.U. per day in 1992. (For comparison, in the U.S. it has been 200 I.U. a day). This reduction in the daily allowance had no scientific basis except the observation that this amount of vitamin D is present in a teaspoonful of cod-liver oil which has long been considered safe and effective in preventing rickets.

In the last decades, the incidence of Type 1 diabetes in Finland has been climbing which is most likely related to the decrease in the daily recommended allowance of vitamin D. As of 1999, Finland has the highest reported incidence of Type 1 diabetes in the world (3). In Finland, the yearly sunshine and therefore vitamin D skin synthesis is much lower compared to more southern areas. Therefore, the population in Finland is at even higher risk for vitamin D deficiency.

Not only in Finland, but in other countries as well, scientists have discovered the amazing power of vitamin D supplementation in preventing Type 1 diabetes. In one such study called EURODIAB (4), researchers found vitamin D supplementation during infancy can significantly reduce the risk for developing Type 1 diabetes. This study was carried out in seven centers in different countries across a variety of populations in Europe.

TYPE 2 DIABETES

Although Type 2 diabetes typically affects adults, recently its incidence among teenagers is on the rise. Type 2 diabetes develops due to insulin resistance, a process in the body that makes it harder for insulin to do its job of keeping blood glucose normal. The body responds to this resistance by producing more and more insulin. After a few years of escalating insulin resistance, the body can't keep up with the huge demands for insulin production. At this point, insulin production starts to decline relative to insulin resistance. Consequently, blood sugar starts to rise.

If your fasting blood glucose rises into the range of 100-125 mg/dl, you have pre-diabetes. When your fasting blood glucose is above 125 mg/dl, you have diabetes. You go through a period of pre-diabetes for many years before you eventually become diabetic.

Because Type 2 diabetes develops gradually, patients typically do not experience the usual diabetes symptoms such as excessive thirst and excessive urination, unless their diabetes remains undiagnosed for a very long period. Type 2 diabetes is usually diagnosed on a routine blood test. For details, please refer to my book, "Take Charge of Your Diabetes."

The Relationship Between Vitamin D Deficiency and Type 2 Diabetes ▪

Is there a relationship between vitamin D deficiency and development of Type 2 diabetes? The answer is yes. Life-style factors that are well known to cause Type 2 diabetes include obesity, old age and physical inactivity. It's interesting to note that all of these factors also cause vitamin D deficiency.

Vitamin D is important for normal glucose metabolism. It acts through several mechanisms on glucose metabolism:

1. Vitamin D directly acts on insulin producing cells in the pancreas to produce more insulin.
2. Vitamin D directly acts on the muscle and fat cells to improve insulin action by reducing insulin resistance.
3. Vitamin D reduces inflammation which is commonly present in patients with Insulin Resistance Syndrome and Type 2 diabetes.
4. Vitamin D indirectly improves insulin production and its action by improving the level of calcium inside the cells.

Now you can understand the important role vitamin D plays in keeping blood glucose normal. Intuitively, vitamin D deficiency can lead to diabetes.

Evidence that Links Vitamin D Deficiency to Type 2 Diabetes ━━━━

Is there any scientific evidence to link vitamin D deficiency to Type 2 diabetes? The answer is yes. Numerous scientific studies have found vitamin D to be low in patients with Type 2 diabetes.

One such remarkable study (5) looked at the level of vitamin D, prevalence of insulin resistance and risk for Type 2 diabetes in the U.S. population. In this study, researchers concluded that people with a low level of vitamin D were at high risk for the development of insulin resistance and Type 2 diabetes.

Evidence that Vitamin D can Prevent Type 2 Diabetes ━━━━

Is there evidence to show that vitamin D can prevent the development of Type 2 diabetes? The answer is yes. In a study (6) from Finland, researchers collected health data in men and women from the ages of 40 to 74. None of these individual had Type 2 diabetes at the start of the study. They followed these individuals for 22 years to see the pattern of development of Type 2 diabetes. These researchers found that people who had higher level of vitamin D were less likely to develop Type 2 diabetes. Thus vitamin D appears to have a protective effect against the development of Type 2 diabetes.

In another study (7) from the U.S., researchers found that vitamin D and calcium supplementation were able to reduce progression from pre-diabetes to diabetes. This protective effect of vitamin D was similar in magnitude to other measures which have been shown to reduce the progression from pre-diabetes to diabetes, such as a weight reducing diet, intense exercise and use of the drug, metformin.

In summary, vitamin D has the potential to prevent Type 1 as well as Type 2 diabetes. It can also prevent the devastating complications of diabetes such as heart attacks and kidney failure. Unfortunately, most diabetics continue to be low in vitamin D. Many diabetics are on a long list of expensive medications, but unfortunately, all too often, vitamin D is not included. Sadly, most physicians don't pay attention to the important relationship between vitamin D and the health of a diabetic patient. Isn't it time that proper vitamin D supplementation become an integral part of diabetes management?

For an in depth, complete discussion of insulin resistance and diabetes, please refer to my book, "Take Charge of Your Diabetes."

REFERENCES:

1. Svoren BM, Volkening LK, Wood JR, Laffel LM. Significant vitamin D deficiency in youth with Type 1 diabetes mellitus. *J Pediatr*.2009;154(1):132-134.

2. Hypponen E, Laara E, Reunanen A, et al. Intake of vitamin D and risk of Type 1 diabetes: a birth-cohort study. *Lancet* 2001;358:1500-1503.

3. Onkamo P, Vaananen S, Karvonen M, Tuomilchto J. Worldwide increase in incidence of Type 1 diabetes: the analysis of the data on published incidence trends. *Diabetologia* 1999;42:1395-1403.

4. The EURODIAB Substudy 2 Study Group. Vitamin D supplementation in early childhood and risk for Type 1 (insulin- dependent) diabetes mellitus. *Diabetologia* 1999;42:51-54.

5. Scragg R, Sowers M, Bell C. Serum 25-hydroxyvitamin D, diabetes, and ethnicity in the third National Health and Nutrition Examination Survey. *Diabetes Care* 2004;(27):28132818.

6. Knekt P, Laaksonen M et al. Serum vitamin D and subsequent occurrence of Type 2 diabetes. *Epidemiology* 2008;(5):666-671.

7. Pittas AG, Harris SS et al. The effects of calcium and vitamin D supplementation on blood glucose and markers of inflammation in non-diabetic adults. *Diabetes Care* 2007;(30):980-986.

CHAPTER 13

Vitamin D Deficiency and High Blood Pressure

High blood pressure, medically known as hypertension, has reached epidemic proportions in the U.S. and around the world. Traditionally, the known risk factors for developing hypertension are: ethnicity, old age, obesity, physical inactivity and stress. Does vitamin D deficiency play any role in the development of hypertension? Scientists wondered. They started to explore this question and were amazed at their findings.

Evidence that Links Vitamin D Deficiency to Hypertension ━━━

In one study (1), scientists discovered that blood pressure was strongly correlated to the distance from the equator. In other words, the farther you lived from the equator, the less vitamin D you obtained from the sun and thus, the higher your blood pressure.

In another study (2), researchers investigated blood pressure differences in individuals of African origin, now living in various parts of the world. They discovered that blood pressure in people of the same ethnicity was higher among those living in northern regions compared to those residing closer to the equator.

In another study (3), scientists investigated blood pressure variations in seasons. They discovered that people living in the same area had higher blood pressure during winter as compared to summer. Less vitamin D from sun exposure during winter was the obvious explanation for higher blood pressure observed during the winter months.

These observational studies led scientists to look deeper at the relationship between vitamin D and blood pressure. In large scale studies (4,5) in the U.S., vitamin D levels were measured in thousands of men and women. In each one of these studies, vitamin D deficiency was found to be an important risk factor for developing hypertension.

How does Vitamin D Deficiency Cause Hypertension? ━━━━

In most people, hypertension develops due to three mechanisms:
- Over-stimulation of a special system in the body, called Renin Angiotensin Aldosterone System (RAAS).
- Insulin resistance.
- Neurogenic mechanism through the "Mind-Body" connection.

1. **Renin Angiotensin Aldosterone System (RAAS)**
   Renin is a chemical in the body which causes production of another chemical, Angiotensin, which in turn raises blood pressure. Angiotensin also stimulates another chemical, called aldosterone, which further raises blood pressure. Aldosterone also reduces potassium in the blood.

   Scientific studies have clearly shown that vitamin D inhibits the RAAS by inhibiting renin. Lack of vitamin D therefore, results in the activation of the RAAS and subsequently, hypertension develops.

2. **Insulin Resistance**

Insulin is a hormone, a chemical in your body, produced by special cells in the pancreas. Insulin then enters the blood stream and exerts its effects on various organs in the body. Due to a variety of reasons, cells in the muscles, fat and liver become resistant to the action of insulin. This is called insulin resistance. In response to insulin resistance, your pancreas produces more and more insulin. These large amounts of insulin cause retention of salt and water by the kidneys and subsequently, your blood pressure becomes elevated.

Vitamin D has been shown to reduce insulin resistance. People deficient in vitamin D lack this beneficial effect and eventually, their insulin resistance worsens, causing an elevation in blood pressure.

Insulin resistance is caused by a variety of factors, vitamin D deficiency being just one of them. Other factors causing insulin resistance are: genetics, obesity, physical inactivity, old age and stress.

Insulin resistance not only causes hypertension, but has various other manifestations which include low HDL (good) cholesterol, pre-diabetes, diabetes, heart disease, stroke, polycystic ovaries and fatty liver.

3. **Neurogenic Mechanism Through the Mind-Body Connection**
   Your blood pressure is also under the control of your brain through the mind-body connection. That's how stress causes an increase in blood pressure. The connection between stress and high blood pressure is now common knowledge. People who are low in vitamin D appear to be more susceptible to depression and that's how vitamin D deficiency may play a role in causing hypertension through the mind-body connection.

Evidence that Vitamin D Can Reduce Blood Pressure ━━━━━

Once scientists clearly recognized the relationship between vitamin D deficiency and high blood pressure, they then wanted to see if blood pressure could be reduced with vitamin D supplementation. In one study (6), researchers gave vitamin D 800 I.U. per day for 6 weeks in elderly women who had vitamin D deficiency. These researchers found that vitamin D supplementation caused a 9% reduction in blood pressure.

In another study (7), patients with mild hypertension were randomly assigned to receive UVB or UVA exposure from a UV lamp three times a week for six weeks. Skin exposure to only UVB (and not UVA) produces vitamin D. Consequently, the blood level of vitamin D rose by 162% in patients receiving UVB. In these patients, blood pressure dropped by 6 mm Hg.; Meanwhile, for those in the UVA group, there was no change in blood pressure.

Vitamin D - A Natural Anti-Hypertensive Agent ━━━━━

Vitamin D is truly a natural anti-hypertensive agent. It is cheap, safe and has many health benefits in addition to lowering high blood pressure. Unfortunately, most physicians are unaware of these facts and don't utilize vitamin D in the treatment of hypertension. Instead, they place patients on expensive drugs with many potential side effects. Even more important, these drugs don't treat the root causes of hypertension, and therefore, sooner or later, more medications are needed to control hypertension. Many people end up on two, three or sometimes even more medications to control their hypertension.

My Approach to Treating Hypertension. ━━━━━

I am not against using medications. I do use drugs to treat hypertension in my patients. However, I also go deeper, educating my patients about the root causes of hypertension, most of which are due to our modern life-style. I guide them towards life-style changes including weight loss, physical activity and stress reduction. I also instruct them about the proper dosage of vitamin D (discussed in detail in Chapter 23, Treatment of Vitamin D Deficiency).

With this approach, most people can control their hypertension with the addition of only one drug, often in small doses. Some can even control mild hypertension without any medication.

When it comes to anti-hypertensive drugs, I most frequently prescribe ACE- inhibitors (Angiotensin Converting Enzyme inhibitors) and ARB (Angiotensin Receptor Blocking) drugs. Both of these classes of drugs act by inhibiting the RAAS. These drugs not only control hypertension, but are also beneficial for the heart as well as the kidneys.

Some examples of ACE-inhibitor drugs are:
Lisinopril (brand Zestril)
Benazepril (brand Lotensin)
Ramipril (brand Altace)
Perindopril (brand Aceon)
Quinapril (brand Accupril)

Some examples of ARB drugs are:
Losartan (brand Cozaar)
Valsartan (brand Diovan)
Irbesartan (brand Avapro)
Candesartan (brand Atacand)
Olmesartan (brand Benicar)

References:

1. Rostand SG. Ultraviolet light may contribute to geographical and racial blood pressure differences. *Hypertension* 1997;(30):150-156.
2. Cooper R, Rotimi C. Hypertensions in populations of West

African Origin: is there a genetic predisposition. *J Hypertens* 1994;12:215-227.

3. Woodhouse PR, Khaw KT, Plummer M. Seasonal variation of blood pressure and its relationship to ambient temperature in an elderly population. *J Hypertens* 1993;11:1267-1274.

4. Forman J, Giovannuci E, et al. Plasma 25-hydroxyvitamin D levels and risk of incidental hypertension. *Hypertension* 2007;(49):1063-1069.

5. Scragg R, Sowers M, Bell C. Serum 25-hydoxyvitamin D, ethnicity, and blood pressure in the Third National Health and Nutrition Examination Survey. *Am J Hypertens* 2007;(7):713-719.

6. Pfeifer M, Begerow B, et al. Effects of a short-term vitamin D(3) and calcium supplementation on blood pressure and parathyroid hormone levels in elderly women. *J Clin Endocrinol Metab* 2001;86:1633-1637.

7. Krause R, Buhring M et al. Ultra-violet B and blood pressure. *Lancet* 1998;(352):709-710.

CHAPTER 14

Vitamin D Deficiency and Kidney Disease

Vitamin D deficiency has a dual relationship to chronic kidney disease.

1. Chronic kidney disease causes vitamin D deficiency.
2. Vitamin D deficiency worsens chronic kidney disease, increasing your odds of ending up on dialysis.

Chronic Kidney Disease Causes Vitamin D Deficiency

Vitamin D deficiency is a common problem in patients with chronic kidney disease. As discussed earlier in Chapter 2, vitamin D is synthesized in the skin. After its production, vitamin D enters the blood stream and reaches the liver where it undergoes a chemical change known as hydroxylation. Hence, vitamin D is converted to 25 (OH) vitamin D (25 hydroxy vitamin D), also called Calcifediol. It re-enters the blood stream and reaches the kidneys where another chemical reaction (hydroxylation) takes place. At that point, 25 (OH) vitamin D is converted to 1,25 $(OH)_2$ vitamin D (or 1,25 dihydroxy vitamin D), also called Calcitriol. It re-enters the blood stream and exerts its biochemical effects. Therefore, Calcitriol is considered the active form of vitamin D.

Now let's examine what happens as a person develops kidney

failure. The conversion of 25 (OH) vitamin D (calcifediol) to 1,25 $(OH)_2$ vitamin D (calcitriol) does not take place properly. Therefore, these patients become low in calcitriol. Chronic kidney disease causes a gradual, but progressive decline in kidney function. Therefore, the formation of calcitriol gradually decreases. This decrease in calcitriol causes a decrease in calcium absorption from the intestines.

However, then a compensatory mechanism kicks in: The parathyroid glands in the neck start to produce a large amount of parathyroid hormone (PTH). This large amount of PTH exerts its effects on the kidneys and enhances the conversion of 25 (OH) vitamin D (calcifediol) into 1,25 $(OH)_2$ vitamin D (calcitriol). But, it comes at a price. The high amount of PTH dissolves calcium from the bones, which then become weakened. In addition, if this compensatory increase in PTH production remains unchecked, patients end up with tumors of the parathyroid glands and a high blood calcium level. For these reasons, patients on End-stage kidney disease are given calcitriol (or its synthetic analogue) supplementation. This prevents the compensatory increase in PTH production and therefore, prevents weakening of bones and tumor formation in the parathyroid glands.

Vitamin D Deficiency Worsens Chronic Kidney Disease, Increasing Your Odds of Ending Up on Dialysis. ▬▬▬▬▬▬▬▬▬

If you recall from Chapter 13, Vitamin D Deficiency and High Blood Pressure, there is a special system in the body called the Renin Angiotensin Aldosterone System (RAAS). Renin is a hormone in the body which causes production of another hormone, Angiotensin, which in turn raises blood pressure. Angiotensin also stimulates another hormone, called aldosterone, which further raises blood pressure. Aldosterone also reduces potassium in the blood. Normal functioning of this (RAAS) system is important in maintaining blood pressure and keeping potassium in the blood in a normal range. However, when your RAAS becomes overactive, high blood pressure (hypertension) develops. *An overactive RAAS and hypertension cause damage to the kidneys and are the main culprits in the progression of kidney disease.*

An overactive RAAS is often seen in people with diabetes and that's why they often have hypertension and kidney disease as well. Currently we use two types of drugs to deal with an overactive RAAS: ACE-inhibitors (Angiotensin Converting Enzyme inhibitors) and ARB (Angiotensin Receptor Blocking) drugs.

Now consider Vitamin D. It inhibits the RAAS by inhibiting renin and therefore, counteracts an overactive RAAS in patients with diabetes, hypertension and chronic kidney disease. Therefore, doesn't it make sense to make sure these patients have a good level of vitamin D?

I utilize ACE inhibitors and/or ARB drugs in my patients with diabetes, hypertension and chronic kidney disease, but I also make sure that these patients have a good level of vitamin D which can also help suppress the RAAS. Unfortunately, most physicians aren't aware of this beneficial effect of vitamin D. Consequently, vitamin D often stays low in patients with hypertension and diabetes. Many patients are not even on ACE inhibitors or ARB drugs. Unfortunately, many of these patients end up with chronic kidney disease. The sad end result is that the kidneys cease to function and they end up on dialysis.

Now you can understand why proper vitamin D supplementation in every patient with diabetes and hypertension is crucial. This simple strategy may help prevent kidney failure as well as incalculable physical, emotional and economic sufferings.

CHAPTER **15**

Vitamin D Deficiency in Stomach Bypass Surgery Patients

Obesity has reached epidemic proportions in the U.S. and around the world. Obesity is the root cause of many serious medical conditions including diabetes, hypertension, cholesterol disorder, heart disease, cancer, gall stones, polycystic ovaries and degenerative arthritis. In most cases, obesity is the result of *overeating*.

Many people are *unable* or *unwilling* to change their eating habits. Therefore, they seek out alternatives. Stomach bypass surgery is one such alternative. In recent years, stomach bypass surgery has become an increasingly common procedure in the U.S. Most people do lose weight with these procedures, but also develop severe vitamin and nutritional deficiencies as well as endocrine abnormalities which often go unrecognized and untreated.

Vitamin D deficiency and secondary hyperparathyroidism are the endocrine abnormalities frequently seen in patients after stomach bypass surgery. Secondary hyperparathyroidism is the result of chronic vitamin D deficiency. Hyperparathyroidism means an increase in parathyroid hormone which dissolves calcium from your bones. Consequently, these patients start to experience generalized body aches and pains. Physicians often place them on pain killers and sometimes even anti-depression medications, while the root cause of their symptoms, vitamin D deficiency, remains undiagnosed and untreated.

I have seen several such cases. After years of going from physician to physician, undergoing expensive diagnostic testing and getting a variety of labels for their symptoms such as Fibromyalgia and Chronic Fatigue Syndrome, these patients are astonished to discover that it all boils down to vitamin D deficiency. Proper vitamin D supplementation takes care of their symptoms. See Chapter 6, Vitamin D Deficiency and Body Aches, Pains and Chronic Fatigue Syndrome, for details on secondary hyperparathyroidism.

CASE STUDY

Jenny, a 63 year old Caucasian female, underwent stomach bypass surgery for obesity. About three years later, I got involved in her medical care. I was surprised to see that she was not taking any vitamin D. She was having a lot of severe aches and pains and was told that she had fibromyalgia.

I ordered her vitamin D level which turned out to be very low. I also ordered her parathyroid hormone which turned out to be very high. Her stomach surgery had caused her to be very low in vitamin D which led to another disease, secondary hyperparathyroidism. That was the reason for her generalized aches and pains.

If you're planning to undergo gastric bypass surgery, ask your doctors to check your 25 (OH) vitamin D level and parathyroid hormone level before surgery. You should go on a good dose of vitamin D before surgery and stay on this dose during your hospital stay and recovery period. (See Chapter 23, Treatment of Vitamin D Deficiency).

You need to be the advocate of your vitamin D supplementation, especially during your hospital stay. Why? Because while you're in the hospital, vitamin D is the last thing on any one's mind. However, you can take care of it by reminding your physician in the hospital. It may actually hasten your recovery.

Afterwards, ask your physician to periodically (about every 3 months) check your 25 (OH) vitamin D level and parathyroid hormone level until you're on a stable dose of vitamin D and your parathyroid hormone is normal. Even after that, continue to have your 25 (OH) vitamin D level checked every 3 months. You should stay diligent about your vitamin D level, as well as other vitamin and mineral supplementation including vitamin B12.

CHAPTER 16

Vitamin D Deficiency and Dental Problems

Vitamin D plays an important role in the health of teeth. Teeth are a form of bone and we know how important vitamin D is for the health of bones. In addition, vitamin D has anti-inflammatory properties and may reduce your risk for periodontal disease.

In a recent study, researchers found that people with a higher level of vitamin D were less likely to have gingivitis (gum inflammation) as compared to people with a low level of vitamin D (1). Findings of this study are in line with my own observations. Ever since I started getting my patient's vitamin D at an optimal level, their dentists have expressed surprise at the great condition of their teeth. They often receive compliments from their dentists.

My own story provides a good illustration. One day about ten years ago, I felt a sharp pain in one of my teeth while I was having lunch. I saw my dentist promptly, who discovered that a molar tooth had fractured. Why? There was no satisfactory answer. My dentist warned me that I was at risk for more dental fractures in the future. Soon afterwards, I got enlightened about vitamin D and started taking vitamin D3, 8000 I.U. a day. No more dental fractures. Actually, my dentist now comments on how strong my teeth are!

REFERENCES:

1. Dietrich T, Nunn M et al. Association between serum concentration of 25-hydroxyvitamin D and gingival inflammation. *Am J Clin Nutr* 2005;82(3):575-580.

CHAPTER **17**

Vitamin D Deficiency and Depression

Can winter blues may be a consequence of vitamin D deficiency? Is there a relationship between low vitamin D and mood disorders? The answer is yes!

Scientific studies (1, 2) have shown that people with mood disorders such as seasonal mood disorder and depression are frequently low in vitamin D. One study (2) even found that older adults with a low vitamin D level, are not only more likely to be depressed, but also may have poor cognitive performance. So, don't blame memory loss simply on getting older. It may the result of low vitamin D as well. Vitamin D deficiency may be a risk factor for Alzheimer's dementia.

Historically, physicians have been unaware of the link between vitamin D deficiency and depression. However, recently some physicians have started to look into the mounting scientific evidence that links vitamin D deficiency to depression.

When I see any individual who has mood disorder such as low mood or depression, I pay particular attention to their vitamin D level. It's almost always low. With proper vitamin D supplementation, I bring their vitamin D level into the optimal range. In my practice, I find these individuals to have more zest for life after proper vitamin D supplementation. Their body aches and pains get less severe and perhaps, that also contributes to their overall sense of well-being.

REFERENCES:

1. Hoogendijk WJ et al. Depression is associated with decreased 25-hydroxyvitamin D and increased parathyroid hormone level in older adults. *Arch Gen Psychiatry.* 2008;65(5):508-512.
2. Wilkins CH et al. Vitamin D deficiency is associated with low mood and worse cognitive performance in older adults. *Am J Geriatr Psychiatry.* 2006;14(12):1032-1040.

CHAPTER 18

Vitamin D Deficiency and Skin Disorders

Skin not only synthesizes vitamin D, but also responds to vitamin D in maintaining its own health. Based on this scientific observation, physicians investigated vitamin D as a therapeutic agent for a skin condition called *psoriasis*. With psoriasis, there's a thickening of the skin in various parts of the body, giving rise to plaques of thick, reddened skin. Researchers were curious if vitamin D treatment could have some beneficial effects on the skin of these individuals. Indeed, their hypothesis was correct.

In one study, researchers found vitamin D as a skin cream to be an effective treatment for a majority of patients with psoriasis (1). This led to the development of a synthetic vitamin D analog called calcipotriene (brand name Dovonex, available as skin cream) which is now commonly used in the treatment of psoriasis.

REFERENCES:

1. Smith EL, Pincus SH, Donovan L, Holick MF. A novel approach for the evaluation and treatment of psoriasis. *J Am Acad Dermatol* 1988;(19):516-519.

CHAPTER 19

Vitamin D Deficiency During Pregnancy and Breastfeeding

A majority of pregnant women are low in vitamin D. Compared to women with fair skin, women with dark skin are even more likely to be vitamin D deficient. According to one recent study (1), 54% of black, pregnant women and 47% of white, pregnant women living in the northern U.S. were low in vitamin D.

Pregnant women who are low in vitamin D are not limited to the U.S. but are a worldwide public health problem. A study from Belgium (2) revealed that 88% of the pregnant women in the area of Liege, Belgium were low in vitamin D. In a study from India (3), researchers found 84% of the pregnant women living in sun-drenched northern India were deficient in vitamin D.

Why are Pregnant Women Low in Vitamin D?

Most women are low in vitamin D before they become pregnant: the problem simply gets worse during pregnancy. Many pregnant women stay indoors for a variety of reasons. Most women feel nauseated during early pregnancy. Later in the pregnancy, there's a lot of discomfort and fatigue. Staying indoors and resting is therefore quite common during pregnancy.

Don't Rely on Prenatal Vitamins for your Vitamin D Needs ━━━

Many pregnant women take a prenatal vitamin assuming it meets all of their vitamin requirements. Think again! Prenatal vitamins contain only a small dose of vitamin D - 400 I.U.; Studies (1, 4) have documented that many pregnant women are low on this dose of vitamin D. My own clinical experience testifies to it.

CASE STUDY

Monika consulted me for her thyroid problem. Later, when she became pregnant, she saw an obstetrician, while I managed her thyroid problem.

I remember the conversation we had when I advised her about vitamin D. "But I've been taking a prenatal vitamin faithfully and it contains 100% of the recommended dose for vitamin D, so I think I should be OK on vitamin D", Monika had replied. I told her we needed to check her vitamin D level just to be safe. Her vitamin D level turned out to be low as 22 ng/ml. She was quite surprised.

The take home message is this: get your vitamin D level checked, even though your prenatal vitamin says that it meets 100% of the daily requirement for vitamin D.

Can Vitamin D Deficiency in the Mother cause Vitamin D Deficiency in the Newborn? ━━━

The answer is yes. The growing fetus derives vitamin D from his/her mother. Therefore, low vitamin D in the mother leads to low vitamin D levels in the fetus. Several studies have found newborns to be low in vitamin D if their mothers were low in vitamin D during pregnancy.

EFFECTS OF VITAMIN D DEFICIENCY ━━━━━━━━━━

Scientific studies show that low vitamin D during pregnancy may jeopardize the health of the mother as well the newborn baby. Studies show the following effects of low vitamin D in pregnant women and their newborns.

Risks to Mother:

1. **High Risk for Gestational Diabetes**

   In the second half of pregnancy, some pregnant women develop gestational diabetes. The known underlying mechanism for gestational diabetes is insulin resistance caused by a variety of factors including placental hormones. Now we know that vitamin D deficiency worsens insulin resistance and therefore, it is intuitive to consider vitamin D deficiency as one of the factors that causes gestational diabetes. In a recent study (5) from Australia, researchers found that pregnant women who were low in vitamin D had an increase in fasting blood glucose, blood insulin level and insulin resistance.

2. **High Risk for Preeclampsia in Pregnant Women**

   Preeclampsia is a serious, potentially life-threatening condition that some women develop during the second half of their pregnancy. When a pregnant woman develops preeclampsia, her blood pressure becomes elevated, the ankles swell up and there is excessive wasting of proteins in the urine. There is a real danger to the life of the mother as well as the baby.

   In an excellent study from Pittsburgh, Pennsylvania (6), researchers found that pregnant women who had low vitamin D had a 5-fold increase in the risk of preeclampsia. Studies have also shown that proper vitamin D supplementation during pregnancy can reduce the risk for hypertension and preeclampsia.

3. Increased Risk for Cesarean Section
   An interesting study (7) recently showed that pregnant women with low level of vitamin D are at high risk for cesarean section. In this study, researchers found that pregnant women who were low in vitamin D were *4 times* more likely to have a cesarean section compared to women with an adequate level of vitamin D.

RISKS TO NEWBORN:

1. **Low Birth Weight**
   Vitamin D plays an important role in the growth of the fetus. Scientific studies have documented that babies born to mothers with low vitamin D level are likely to have low birth weight.

2. **Rickets and Soft Skull Bones (Craniotabes) at Birth**
   Vitamin D plays a vital role in the development of fetal bones. Deficiency of vitamin D can cause a delay in the maturation of the bones and can result in rickets and craniotabes. Rickets typically causes deformity of the bones of the legs, chest wall and generalized weakness of muscles.

   Craniotabes refers to soft skull bones at birth. It's diagnosed if the examiner's fingers can bend skull bones, which then pop back after pressure is released. It's also called "ping-pong ball skull." Craniotabes can affect up to 30% of otherwise normal newborns. It is presumed to spontaneously heal in most cases by 2-3 months. This has led to the notion (without any scientific background) that physicians need not pay much attention to this condition.

   What is the cause of craniotabes? Japanese researchers investigated and found the answer: vitamin D deficiency! In an excellent study (8) from Japan, researchers found that the incidence of craniotabes was inversely related to sun exposure during the last *four* months of pregnancy. Incidence was highest if delivery took place during spring because the pregnant mother had less exposure to the sun during the preceding winter. The incidence of craniotabes was lowest if delivery took place in fall because the pregnant mothers had more sun exposure during the preceding summer.

They also checked vitamin D, parathyroid hormone and x-rays of the hand in infants with craniotabes at one month of age. The results were amazing. Vitamin D level turned out to be low in the vast majority (over 90%) of these infants. More than one third even had early rickets. Those who were solely breast fed without any formula (formula contains vitamin D) had even lower levels of vitamin D. Ten percent of these infants even had secondary hyperparathyroidism.

3. **Decreased Bone Mass in Childhood**
   Vitamin D is extremely important for the health of the bones. Vitamin D starts playing this vital role before you are born, while you are still in the uterus. The effects of low vitamin D on the fetus not only make bones weak at birth, but also appears to continue to adversely affect bones for the rest of childhood and perhaps adult life as well.

   In a study (9), researchers from the U.K. followed children born to women with low vitamin D and measured their bone mass at age 9. The researchers were amazed to find that children with low vitamin D level at birth had low bone mass at age 9 compared to those children who did not suffer from vitamin D deficiency at birth. It appears that vitamin D deficiency during fetal development has long term negative effects on the health of the bones.

4. Asthma and Type 1 Diabetes during Childhood.

Vitamin D plays an important role in the development of the immune system of the fetus. Therefore, newborns low in vitamin D are at increased risk for autoimmune diseases such as Type 1 diabetes and asthma.

In one study from Boston (10), researchers found that vitamin D intake of pregnant women had an inverse relationship with the development of asthma in their child. In this study, pregnant women taking a higher dose of vitamin D of about 800 I.U. a day, significantly reduced the risk of developing asthma in their child compared to women taking a lower dose of about 400 I.U. a day.

In another study, researchers from Finland (11) found infants who received a large daily dose of vitamin D (2000 I.U. per day) had an amazing 80% risk reduction for the development of Type 1 diabetes during childhood and early adulthood.

5. Maternal Vitamin D Deficiency can also cause other medical problems in infants. These include under-developed teeth, congestive heart failure, low blood calcium and tetany. Tetany refers to involuntary spasms of muscles.

In summary, maternal vitamin D deficiency leads to deficiency of vitamin D in the fetus. Vitamin D deficiency poses risks to the health of the mother as well as the newborn. Moreover, it appears that the imprints of vitamin D deficiency during fetal life persists throughout childhood and perhaps even into adult life and contributes to a number of chronic illnesses such as asthma, Type 1 diabetes and weak bones.

Therefore, by simply ensuring a good level of vitamin D during pregnancy and infancy, you can give your offspring a healthy start in life.

Low Vitamin D in Breast-fed Infants ━━━━━━━━

Women who breastfeed their infants need more calcium because calcium is an important ingredient of milk. Therefore, they need more vitamin D because vitamin D is vital in the absorption of calcium from the intestines.

Breast milk has very little vitamin D. Therefore, women who breastfeed their infant must take a good dose of vitamin D themselves (see Chapter 23, Treatment of Vitamin D Deficiency) and also give their baby at least a daily dose of 400 I.U. of vitamin D.

Most pediatricians know that human milk is very low in vitamin D. However, what many pediatricians may not know is that low vitamin D in human milk is a reflection of low vitamin D in the lactating mother. It was brilliantly pointed out in a recent study (12). The researchers showed that the milk of lactating women who had adequate level of vitamin D contained vitamin D equal to the amount contained in infant formula.

"So, What Should I Do?" ━━━━━━━━

Get your vitamin D level checked if you plan to get pregnant. Try to get your vitamin D at a good level even before pregnancy. Continue proper vitamin D supplementation during and after pregnancy. Have your vitamin D level checked at least every 2 months during and after your pregnancy. Please note that if you breastfeed your baby, you need even more vitamin D supplementation. For details, please refer to Chapter 23, Treatment of Vitamin D Deficiency.

REFERENCES:

1. Bodnar LM, Simhan HN et al. High prevalence of vitamin D insufficiency in black and white pregnant women residing in the northern United States and their neonates. *J Nutr.* 2007;137:447-452.

2. Cavalier E, Delanaye P, et al. Vitamin D deficiency in recently pregnant women. *Rev Med Liege.* 2008;63(2):87-91.

3. Sachan A, Gupta R, et al. High prevalence of vitamin D deficiency among pregnant women and their new-borns in northern India. *Am J Clin Nutr.* 2005;81:1060-1064.

4. Lee JM, Smith JR, et al. Vitamin D deficiency in a healthy group of mothers and newborn infants. *Clin Pediatr.* 2007;46:42-44.

5. Clifton-Bligh RJ, McElduff P, McElduff A. Maternal vitamin D deficiency, ethnicity and gestational diabetes. *Diabet Med.* 2008;25(6):678-684.

6. Bodnar L, Catov J, et al. Maternal vitamin D deficiency increases the risk of preeclampsia. *J Clin Endocrinol Metab.* 2007;92(9):3517-3522.

7. Merewood A, Mehta SD, et al. Association between vitamin D deficiency and primary cesarean section. *J Clin Endocrinol Metab.* 2009;94(3):940-945.

8. Yorifuji J, Yorifuji T, et al. Craniotabes in normal newborns: the earliest sign of subclinical vitamin D deficiency. *J Clin Endocrinol Metab.* 2008;93(5):1784-1788.

9. Javaid MK et al. Maternal vitamin D status during pregnancy and childhood bone mass at 9 years: a longitudinal study. *Lancet.* 2006;367(9504):36-43.

10. Camargo jr C, Rifas-Shiman S, et al. Maternal intake of vitamin D during pregnancy and risk of recurrent wheezing in children at 3 y of age. *Am J Clin Nutr* 2007;85:788-795.

11. Hypponen E, Laara E, Reunanen A, et al. Intake of vitamin D and risk of Type 1 diabetes: a birth-cohort study. *Lancet* 2001;358:1500-1503.

12. Taylor SN, Wagner CL, Hollis BW. Vitamin D supplementation during lactation to support infant and mother. *J Am Coll Nutr.* 2008;27(6):690-701.

CHAPTER 20

Vitamin D Deficiency in Children and Teenagers

Vitamin D deficiency is common among children and teenagers. Unfortunately, it remains undiagnosed and untreated. Consequences of vitamin D deficiency during childhood include rickets, decrease in overall strength of bones, a defective immune system, frequent colds, asthma, inflammatory bowel disease, Type 1 diabetes and dental problems.

Vitamin D Deficiency is Common among Children ━━━━━━

In a study (1) reported in 2008 in the *Archives of Pediatrics & Adolescent Medicine*, researchers noted vitamin D level to be low in 40% of infants and toddlers. They also noted X-rays changes of rickets in 7.5% and weak bones in 32% of infants and toddlers in this study. These were otherwise healthy children, attending primary care clinics in the U.S. This certainly contradicts the belief that rickets doesn't exist in the U.S. anymore. In another study (2) published in 2008, researchers reported vitamin D to be low in 74% of obese children and adolescents in the Wisconsin area.

Vitamin D deficiency is not limited to the U.S. and Europe, but is a global phenomenon. It's reported to be prevalent in sunny countries such as New Zealand as well as countries in the Middle East.

Causes for Vitamin D Deficiency in Children ━━━━━━━━

Vitamin D deficiency does not spare children of any geographic location or any race or ethnicity.

However, the following factors do make children and teenagers more susceptible to vitamin D deficiency:

1. **Less exposure to the sun** for a variety of reasons including:
   A. *Sun phobia among parents.* Avoidance of sun exposure as well as high usage of   sunscreen when outside.
   B. *Cultural customs* (very prevalent in certain countries) to cover most of the body with clothing.
   C. *High latitudes* such as in Canada, the Northeastern U.S. and the U.K.

2. **Infants who are solely breast-fed** as breast milk contains only negligible amounts of vitamin D. Among toddlers, low milk consumption contributes to vitamin D deficiency.

3. **Skin pigmentation** decreases the skin's ability to synthesize vitamin D from sun exposure. Therefore, children of African American, Asian and Hispanic descent are even more likely to have vitamin D deficiency.

4. **Obesity** is another important factor that causes vitamin D deficiency. Because vitamin D is fat soluble, fat traps vitamin D. Therefore, less vitamin D is available for the rest of the body.

5. **Certain medical conditions** such as malabsorption, chronic kidney disease and anti-epilepsy drugs can further lower vitamin D level.

Effects of Vitamin D Deficiency in Children ━━━━━━━

1. **RICKETS**

   Severe vitamin D deficiency during childhood causes bones to be so weak that they become deformed. In medical terms, it's called Rickets. In addition, these children also have stunted growth, a deformed chest, muscle weakness and bone pains.

   Rickets, once thought to have been almost eradicated in the U.S., has re-emerged. Cases of rickets are being reported from states in the north such as Massachusetts and Alaska, but also from sunny states such as Texas and California.

   Rickets is being reported all over the world, from countries such as the U.K., India, Bangladesh and several countries in the Middle East.

2. **DECREASED MUSCLE STRENGTH**

   Vitamin D is important for the health of muscles. Low vitamin D can lead to muscle weakness. In a study from the U.K. (3), researchers found vitamin D level to have a direct correlation with muscle strength among teenagers. The higher the vitamin D, the better the muscle strength; the lower the vitamin D, the lower the muscle strength.

3. **DECREASED BONE STRENGTH**

   During childhood and especially during teenage years, you're building your bones. Vitamin D plays a crucial role in building strong bones. This is because vitamin D is important for the absorption of calcium and phosphorus from the intestines and then in incorporating calcium and phosphorus into the bones. Vitamin D deficiency exerts its deleterious effects on the bones.

A study from Finland (4) showed that 62% of adolescent girls were severely low in vitamin D during winter. These otherwise healthy girls had a significant decrease in bone strength as measured by a DXA (Dual energy X-ray Absorptiometry) machine.

In a study from China (5), researchers found that 58% of adolescent girls were low in vitamin D level. Low vitamin D status was associated with low bone density and low muscle strength.

In a study from Ireland (6), researchers found that low vitamin D status adversely affected the bone density of adolescent girls. Those with a good level of vitamin D had stronger bones.

4. HIGH RISK FOR OSTEOPOROSIS

You achieve most of your bone strength (technically called bone density) during adolescence. By the approximate age of twenty five, most of your bone density is achieved. Technically, we call it peak bone density. From here onwards, bone density starts to decline. In later years of life, bone density may decrease to a point where bones can fracture very easily after a trivial trauma. This is called osteoporosis.

It's crucial to achieve a good bone density during adolescence. If vitamin D is low during adolescence, you'll have sub-optimal peak bone strength and suffer from osteoporosis at an earlier age.

5. DENTAL PROBLEMS

Teeth are a form of bone. Vitamin D plays an important role in the health of your teeth. While brushing your teeth is a good thing, don't forget about vitamin D.

6. DEFECTIVE IMMUNE SYSTEMS

As discussed in earlier in Chapter 9, Vitamin D Deficiency and Immune System Diseases, vitamin D is essential to keep the immune system functioning normally. Vitamin D deficiency leads to a defective immune system. Consequently, children low in vitamin D are at increased risk for frequent colds, asthma, inflammatory bowel disease, multiple sclerosis and Type 1 diabetes.

My Recommendations to Parents of Children and Teenagers ━━━

Don't let your child miss the opportunity of building strong bones!
Sensible sun exposure and vitamin D supplement

Most children and teenagers, like the rest of society, often use sunscreen whenever they are outdoors. Therefore, they get hardly any vitamin D from the sun. If your child doesn't have a history of cancer caused by the sun or any other medical reason to avoid the sun, you should probably let your child be outdoors without sunscreen for about 15-30 minutes a day (if skin is fair) or 30-60 minutes (if skin is dark). However, ask your child's health care provider if this amount of sun exposure is appropriate for your child.

In addition, encourage your child to take a vitamin D3 supplement every day. The appropriate amount of vitamin D for your child depends on their size.

DAILY DOSE OF VITAMIN D FOR CHILDREN AND TEENAGERS ━━━

For children (2 months to 10 years): A daily dose of 400-1000 I.U. of vitamin D3.

For teenagers (10 – 19): A daily dose of 1000-2000 I.U. of vitamin D3.

> 1000 I.U. for thin children.
> 2000 I.U. for obese children.

Two other important factors in this regard are good calcium intake and weight bearing exercises. Dairy products such as milk, cheese and yogurt are good sources of calcium. Weight bearing exercises include power (fast) walking, jogging and running. So go outdoors, jog, run and play real sports such as soccer, basketball and tennis. Have fun and build strong bones at the same time.

REFERENCES:

1. Gordon CM, Feldman HA, et al. Prevalence of vitamin D deficiency among healthy infants and toddlers. *Arch Pediatr Adolesc Med*. 2008;162:505-512.
2. Alemzadeh R, Kichler J. Hypovitaminosis D in obese children and adolescents: relationship with adiposity, insulin sensitivity, ethnicity, and season. *Metabolism*. 2008;57(2):183-191.
3. Ward KA, Das G et al. Viatmin D status and muscle function in post-menarchal adolescent girls. *J Clin Endocrinol Metab* 2009;94(2):559-563.
4. Outila TA, Karkkainen MU et al. Vitamin D status affects serum parathyroid hormone concentration during winter in female adolescents: association with forearm bone mineral density. *Am J Clin Nutr*. 2001;74(2):206-210.
5. Foo LH, Zhang O et al. Low vitamin D status has an adverse influence on bone mass, bone turnover and muscle strength in Chinese adolescent girls. *J Nutr*. 2009;139(5):1002-1007.
6. Cashman K, Hill T: Low vitamin D status adversely affects bone health parameters in adolescents. *Am J Clin Nutr*. 2008; 87:1039-1044.

CHAPTER 21

Vitamin D Deficiency in the Elderly

Vitamin D deficiency is rampant among the elderly. In one study (1) from the U.S., researchers found that 72% of older men were low in Vitamin D. What's alarming is that most of these men were taking vitamin D supplements. The level of vitamin D was particularly low among obese, sedentary men living in northern states, especially during winter months.

Causes of Vitamin D Deficiency in the Elderly:

1. **Less sun exposure**
   In general, the elderly spent most of their time indoors due to medical illnesses and physical limitation, such as arthritis and heart disease. Often they end up in hospitals and nursing homes. Vitamin D is the last thing on anyone's mind. A study from Iceland (2) reported that 72% of elderly patients (men and women) in the hospital were low in vitamin D.

2. **Aging causes thinning of the skin.**
   Thin skin is much less capable of synthesizing vitamin D than the thick skin of a young person.

3. **Inadequate level of Vitamin D in multivitamins.**
   Vitamin D present in most multivitamins is usually 400-600

I.U. per day, which is inadequate. That's why these individuals continue to be low in vitamin D despite taking vitamin D supplements.

4. Abdominal Illnesses

The elderly often suffer from a variety of abdominal illnesses which further impair the absorption of vitamin D. These illnesses include Ulcerative Colitis, Crohn's disease and partial resection of the pancreas, stomach or intestines.

5. Some medications interfere with the absorption of vitamin D.

Older patients are more likely to take medications which interfere with the absorption of vitamin D. These medications include:

A. Phenytoin (brand name Dilatin),

B. Phenobarbital

C. Rifampin

D. Orlistat (brand names Xenical and Alli)

E. Cholestyramine (brand names Questran, LoCholest and Prevalite)

F. Steroids. In particular, steroids can cause a severe deficiency of vitamin D.

6. Chronic Kidney Insufficiency

Most elderly patients suffer from some degree of chronic kidney insufficiency caused by aging itself and also due to diseases such as diabetes, hypertension and hardening of the arteries. These individuals are low in vitamin D to start with. In addition, now they become less efficient in converting vitamin D into its active form, $1, 25 (OH)_2$ vitamin D. Double whammy!

Effects of Low Vitamin D ━━━━━━━━━

1. Fatigue

Low vitamin D is one major cause of fatigue that most elderly people experience. In a study (3), researchers from the University of Maryland in Baltimore found a direct association between low vitamin D level and weakness and exhaustion among men 65 years or older.

2. Body aches and pains

Vitamin D deficiency is a major cause of body aches and pains in the elderly. Low vitamin D can lead to secondary hyperparathyroidism which then results in body aches and pains. For details, see Chapter 6, Vitamin D Deficiency and Body Aches, Pains and Chronic Fatigue Syndrome.

3. Osteoporosis

Vitamin D plays a pivotal role in the health of your bones. Low vitamin D leads to weakening of bones, which is technically called osteopenia (early stage) or osteoporosis (more advanced stage).

4. Falls

Vitamin D is important for the health of muscles, joints and bones. Vitamin D deficiency in the elderly causes muscles and bones to weaken. In addition, the elderly often have arthritis. Consequently, they can easily fall and fracture their bones, which can have devastating effects on the quality of life at this age.

5. Heart disease

Vitamin D deficiency increases your odds of having coronary heart disease. For details, see Chapter 11, Vitamin D Deficiency and Heart Disease. An epidemic of coronary heart disease in the elderly may in part be due to the epidemic of vitamin D deficiency.

6. High Blood Pressure (Hypertension)

Vitamin D deficiency is known to increase blood pressure by activating the Renin Angiotensin Aldosterone System (RAAS). For details, see Chapter 13 on Vitamin D Deficiency and High Blood Pressure (Hypertension). Most elderly are low in vitamin D and also have high blood pressure. The correlation is pretty obvious. Hypertension in the elderly may at least in part be due to vitamin D deficiency.

7. Diabetes

Almost all elderly with diabetes have Type 2 diabetes which is caused by a process in your body called insulin resistance. Vitamin D deficiency worsens insulin resistance and thus, may contribute towards development of diabetes.

8. Cancer

Most elderly perhaps fear cancer the most, as it's so prevalent in old age. Vitamin D deficiency may increase the risk for cancer, especially cancers of the colon, breast and prostate, three major cancers of old age. For more information see Chapter 10, Vitamin D Deficiency and Cancer.

9. Depression and Memory Loss

Depression and memory loss are two extremely common problems in the old age. Vitamin D deficiency probably plays some role in causing depression as well as memory loss. For more information, see Chapter 17, Vitamin D Deficiency and Depression.

"What should I do?" ━━━━━━━━━━━━━

Perhaps now you understand the importance of vitamin D in *preventing* so many afflictions in the elderly. Even if you have one of these conditions, proper vitamin D supplementation can help a great deal. For details, please refer to Chapters 22 and 23, Diagnosis and Treatment of Vitamin D Deficiency.

REFERENCES:

1. Orwoll E, Nielson CM et al. Vitamin D deficiency in older men. *J Clin Endocrinol Metab.* 2009;94(4):1214-1222.
2. Ramel A, Jonsson PV, et al. Vitamin D deficiency and nutritional status in elderly hospitalized subjects in Iceland. *Public Health Nutr.* 2009;(7):1001-1005.
3. Shardell M, Hicks GE et al. Association between low vitamin D levels with frailty syndrome in men and women. *J Gerntol A Biol Sci Med Sci* 2009; 64(1):69-75.

CHAPTER 22

Diagnosis of Vitamin D Deficiency

It's easy to diagnose vitamin D deficiency: It's a simple blood test. That's all! However, it needs to be the right test and must be interpreted properly! And that's where a lot of problems arise.

What's the Right Test to Diagnose Vitamin D Deficiency and Why? ▬

Laboratories offer two tests to determine vitamin D level in the blood. In vitamin D deficiency, one of them is low whereas the other one is often normal. Most physicians don't know the distinction between these two tests and may order the wrong test. Consequently, they may say your vitamin D level is normal, when it's actually low.

The right blood test to evaluate your vitamin D status is: <u>25 (OH) vitamin D (25-hydroxy vitamin D).</u>
The other blood test for vitamin D is 1,25 (OH)$_2$ vitamin D (1,25 dihydroxy vitamin D).
This is the wrong test to diagnose vitamin D deficiency! Why?

There are two reasons why 25 (OH) vitamin D and **not** 1,25 (OH)$_2$ vitamin D is the right test to diagnose vitamin D deficiency.

Reason 1:

25 (OH) vitamin D stays in your blood for a much longer period of time (half life of about 3 weeks) compared to 1,25 $(OH)_2$ vitamin D (half life of about 14 hours).

Therefore, 25 (OH) vitamin D more accurately reflects the status of vitamin D in your body.

Reason 2:

As vitamin D deficiency develops, your body increases production of parathyroid hormone by the parathyroid glands situated in your neck. Parathyroid hormone increases the conversion of 25 (OH) vitamin D into 1,25 $(OH)_2$ vitamin D. Consequently, 1,25 $(OH)_2$ vitamin D level in the blood will stay in the normal range (and can even be high) even if you're low in 25 (OH) vitamin D.

<u>CASE STUDY</u>

Jenny, a 63 years old Caucasian female got her vitamin D testing done. The tests included 1,25 $(OH)_2$ vitamin D as well as 25 (OH) vitamin D.

Her 1,25 $(OH)_2$ vitamin D turned out to be high as 72 pg/ml (reference range 15-55 pg/ml).

Her 25 (OH) vitamin D level was extremely low as 5 ng/ml (30- 100 ng/ml).

Her parathyroid hormone level was markedly elevated as 571 pg/ml (reference 12-65 pg/ml).

Her diagnosis was secondary hyperparathyroidism due to severe vitamin D deficiency. If she only had the 1,25 $(OH)_2$ vitamin D level done, her diagnosis of severe vitamin D deficiency would have been missed because her 1,25 $(OH)_2$ vitamin D was not low, but high.

Her 1,25 $(OH)_2$ vitamin D level was high due to her high level of parathyroid hormone which converted 25 (OH)

---

vitamin D into 1,25 (OH)$_2$ vitamin D. In fact, she was very low in vitamin D as was accurately demonstrated by her very low level of 25 (OH) vitamin D.

Interpretation of the Lab Test

To complicate matters further, the normal range reported by most laboratories for vitamin D is outdated and incorrect. Most physicians unfortunately simply interpret a blood test in reference to the "normal range" provided by the lab.

Consequently, physicians may incorrectly advise their patients that their vitamin D level is fine, even when it's not.

Why are the normal ranges for 25 (OH) vitamin D inaccurate?

The normal ranges for vitamin D come from the era when our concern was just to prevent rickets. A small dose of vitamin D is enough to prevent rickets. Therefore, a level of 25 (OH) vitamin D of 10 ng/ml (25 nmol/L) or above was established as adequate to prevent rickets. That's why many laboratories report 10 ng/ml (25 nmol/L) as the lower limit of the normal range.

However, in recent years our understanding of the effects of vitamin D has dramatically changed. Now we understand that vitamin D can do much more than simply prevent rickets. In fact, vitamin D is crucial for maintaining many vital functions in the body, such as a healthy immune system and a healthy heart. In addition, an adequate level of vitamin D may prevent diabetes, osteoporosis and cancer, as discussed earlier.

To achieve these goals, many experts in the field (including myself) recommend a level of 25 (OH) vitamin D to be at least 30 ng/ml (75 nmol/L) and preferably above 50 ng/ml (125 nmol/L). An excellent review of scientific studies (1) published in the *American Journal of*

Clinical Nutrition in 2006 concluded that the most beneficial blood level of 25 (OH) vitamin D starts at 30 ng/ml (or 75 nmol/L).

Unfortunately many laboratories continue to report a normal range with the lower limit of 10 ng/ml (25 nmol/L). Now imagine the following scenario: Your 25 (OH) vitamin D level is19 ng/ml.; Your physician interprets this as normal because it's in the "normal range" provided by the laboratory. However, you are actually quite low in vitamin D! This happens all too frequently.

Watch out for the units used by the Laboratory. ━━━━━━

There is another problem that many physicians are unaware of. Different laboratories report vitamin D level in different units. In the U.S. and around the world, most laboratories report 25 (OH) vitamin D in one of two ways: either as ng/ml or nmol/L.

The conversion factor from ng/ml to nmol/L is about 2.5. For example, if your level is 30 **ng/ml**, you multiply it by 2.5 and will get a number of 75 in **nmol/L**. The lower limit of normal for 25 (OH) vitamin D should be **30 ng/ml or 75 nmol/L**.

Now, let's assume that you are fortunate enough to have a physician who keeps up with the latest information and is proactive about vitamin D supplementation. From attending conferences and reading articles on vitamin D, your physician may simply remember that the lower limit of normal for 25 (OH) vitamin D is 30 (and that's how most physicians remember - just the numbers, without paying attention to the units).

Here's another treacherous case scenario: Your laboratory reports your 25 (OH) vitamin D to be 40 **nmol/L**. Your physician simply looks at the number 40 and tells you your vitamin D is good. In his mind, it's more than 30, so you're fine. In fact, your vitamin D is low because in reality, a level of 40 **nmol/L** is equal to 16 **_ng/ml.!!_** He totally forgot to look closely at the units.

Also, note that the upper limit of normal as reported by many laboratories is also inaccurate. The upper limit of normal should be 100 ng/ml (250 nmol/L).

REFERENCE:

1. Bischoff-Ferrari H et al. Current recommended vitamin D may not be optimal. *Am J Clin Nutr.* 2006;84:18-28.

CHAPTER 23

Treatment of Vitamin D Deficiency

Most physicians do not know how to properly treat vitamin D deficiency. Why? Because it's not taught during their medical training. Nor do they have much experience in their clinical practice. It's a new field for them.

What amazes me is the advice given in newspaper articles, such as "Experts recommend either 400 units of vitamin D a day or 15 minutes of sunshine a day is enough to get a good level of vitamin D." I believe these recommendations are flawed.

Why are Recommendations on the Daily Dose of Vitamin D Flawed? ▬

I check vitamin D level in all of my patients. The majority turn out to be low in vitamin D. Many of them take the recommended dose of 400 I.U. of vitamin D a day. Many of them also go out in the sun at least 15 minutes a day in sunny southern California, yet they're still low in vitamin D. Based on this kind of sound clinical evidence, it's clear to me that 400 I.U. of vitamin D a day is insufficient. Fifteen minutes of sunshine a day is also insufficient to get a good level of vitamin D.

Many scientific studies have clearly demonstrated that the current recommended dose of 400 I.U. of vitamin D per day is not optimal. An excellent review of these studies was published in 2006 in the *American Journal of Clinical Nutrition*. The authors concluded that the beneficial blood level of 25 (OH) vitamin D starts at 30 ng/ml (or 75 nmol/L) and these levels of vitamin D can not be achieved in most patients with the current recommended dose of vitamin D (1).

It's also unscientific to make general recommendations about how much sun exposure can provide you with enough vitamin D. Why? As discussed earlier in Chapter 4 , Natural Sources of Vitamin D, there are many variables that determine vitamin D level in your body including:

1. Latitude

In areas north of 44 degrees N latitude, sun rays are less effective in producing vitamin D in the skin during winter months. The farther north you live, the less effective skin synthesis of vitamin D is from sun exposure.

2. Season

In the same region, the sun is less intense during winter months. Consequently, skin synthesis of vitamin D decreases during wintertime.

3. Age

As you grow older, the skin becomes less efficient in synthesizing vitamin D from sun exposure.

4. Skin Color

The darker your skin, the less efficient it is in forming vitamin D from sun exposure.

5. Sun screens

If you use sunscreen (like most people in the U.S.), then your skin can't form vitamin D, even if you live in a sunny area like Los Angeles or Miami.

6. Lifestyle

Obviously, if you stay out of the sun, you can't form vitamin D in your skin. Many people work indoors and choose leisure activities that are indoors. Similarly, if you cover your entire skin due to cultural reasons (like many women in the Middle-East), you can't form vitamin D from your skin, even though you live in a sunny place.

With so many variables determining vitamin D level, how could "spending 15 minutes a day in the sun" be an accurate recommendation? For example, a New Yorker spending 15 minutes a day in the sun will have a different vitamin D level than a Texan. Even in New York, a person with fair skin will have a different vitamin D level than a person with dark skin. A teenager will have a different level than a grandparent. The same New Yorker will have a different level of vitamin D during summer versus winter. You can see why the "15 minutes of sunshine a day recommendation" is flawed. The "one size fits all" approach doesn't work with an issue that has so many variables!

My Approach to the Treatment of Vitamin D Deficiency ━━━━

Over the last ten years, I've treated thousands of patients with vitamin D deficiency. Based on my own clinical observations, I've developed a unique, scientific yet practical treatment approach that works well for my patients.

1. Assess Vitamin D Status

First of all, I assess and treat every person on an individual basis. I order a 25 (OH) Vitamin D level in the blood to assess vitamin D status. This accurately reflects the impact of variables in life style such as geographic location, season, ethnicity, working habits, eating habits, outdoor activities and sunscreen application habits. No guess work. No blind recommendations. To me, this is the most scientific approach in determining one's vitamin D status!

2. Aim for an optimal level of Vitamin D.

After the lab test, I discuss the results with my patients. As I wrote earlier, the level of 25 (OH) vitamin D should be at least 30 ng/ml (75 nmol/L). Now you may ask, "But what is the optimal level of vitamin D?" Based on my extensive experience, I believe <u>the optimal blood level of 25 (OH) vitamin D to be in the range of 50-100 ng/ml (125-250 nmol/L)</u>. I feel that a vitamin D concentration at this level is important in order to build strong bones, improve immune function, treat aches, pains, chronic fatigue and prevent and treat cancer, heart disease, osteoporosis, tooth fractures, diabetes, high blood pressure, kidney disease and depression.

3. How to achieve a good level of vitamin D

I discuss with each individual patient how to achieve an optimal level of vitamin D.
<u>You can get vitamin D from four sources</u>:
A. Sun exposure
B. Diet
C. Vitamin D supplements
D. Ultraviolet lamps

<u>*For an average person, it's impossible to get a good level of vitamin D from sun exposure or diet alone.*</u> For example, according to my experience, a Caucasian person needs to be out in the sun in southern California in a bathing suit for approximately two to four hours a day to get a good level of vitamin D. Now how many people

can have that kind of lifestyle year round?

In my extensive experience of diagnosing and treating Vitamin D deficiency, I encountered only one person with a good blood level of 25 (OH) vitamin D (above 50 ng/ml without taking any supplements). She was a lifeguard with fair skin who spent about four hours a day, five days a week in the sun in her bathing suit. This amount of sun exposure is not only impractical, but also inadvisable. This degree of sun exposure significantly increases your risk for skin cancer, especially if you have fair skin.

Now consider this: One 8 ounce cup of milk has only 100 I.U. of vitamin D. You'd have to drink 20 - 40 cups a day to get a good level of vitamin D. It's not only impractical, but also inadvisable. Imagine all the calories, the amount of LDL (bad) cholesterol and the natural sugar you'd get from such a huge amount of milk.

A serving of cereal fortified with vitamin D has about 40-80 I.U. of vitamin D. You can imagine how much cereal you'd have to eat to get a good level of vitamin D. There are many negative consequences to eating such a large amount of cereal.

From a practical stand point, I recommend taking advantage of three sources of vitamin D: sun, diet and vitamin D supplements. I never resort to ultraviolet lamps, which are expensive and in my experience, unnecessary.

THE THREE SOURCES OF VITAMIN D ━━━━━━━━━━

1. Sun exposure

Sun is an excellent source of vitamin D, but it can also cause skin cancer. Various physicians make extreme recommendations on sun exposure, depending upon their specialty. Dermatologists, with their tunnel vision, exaggerate the fear of skin cancer and recommend avoiding the sun as much as possible. And don't forget to put on sunscreen each time you go outside! On the other hand, physicians solely interested in vitamin D, with their tunnel vision, recommend liberal sun exposure and minimize the fear of skin cancer. In my opinion, both have myopic views, which unfortunately is a basic flaw inherent to modern medicine. Physicians think in the narrow range of their own specialty and don't consider the overall whole outlook for the patient.

My Recommendations about Sun Exposure

Living in the modern world, you can't obtain a good level of vitamin D simply from sun exposure. However, you should try to get some of your vitamin D from the sun.

Here's my sensible approach to sun exposure:
- People with dark skin, without any history of skin cancer, should spend about 60 minutes a day in the sun, without any sunscreen, between 10 am and 3 pm. If weather permits, try not to cover your arms or your legs below the knees.
- People with fair skin, without any history of skin cancer, should go out in the sun for short periods, about 10 -15 minutes a day, without any sunscreen, between 10 am and 3 pm.
- The duration of sun exposure can be a bit more during winter months and a little less during summer months.
- People with a history of skin cancer should avoid the sun as much as possible and wear sunscreen when they are outdoors.

2. Diet

Diet is not a good source of vitamin D. However, you can get some vitamin D from diet. Please note that when you select food, vitamin D should not be the only consideration. You need to take a more comprehensive approach when selecting food, paying attention to overall ingredients.

Different people have different nutritional requirements, depending on numerous factors such as age, genetics, weight, metabolism, physical activity, seasonal variation and medical conditions such as diabetes, cholesterol disorder, high blood pressure, heart disease, metabolic syndrome, menopause symptoms, polycystic ovary syndrome, thyroid disorders and other medical conditions.

As I mentioned earlier, modern medicine suffers from "narrow mindedness" in the sense that every expert gives advice according to his/her specialty without looking at the overall person as a whole. That's why there are so many different diets, each conflicting with the other, each claiming to be better than the other.

Consider this scenario: In a magazine article, an expert recommends drinking plenty of orange juice because it contains 100 I.U. of vitamin D per cup. So you start drinking a lot of orange juice without realizing that you're also consuming large quantities of sugar and potassium in the orange juice. If you happen to be diabetic, your glucose values will go through the roof. If you have Metabolic Syndrome and are pre-diabetic, your insulin level will skyrocket. If you're an elderly person with diabetes, high blood pressure and kidney failure, your blood sugar will shoot up and your blood potassium may also become elevated, which if not diagnosed and treated appropriately, can be life threatening. As you can see, you can get in a real mess just because you were myopically focusing on improving your vitamin D level.

So, please beware of all ingredients in a food, not just its vitamin D content.

With this understanding, let us take a closer look at some foods and their vitamin D contents:

MILK

Natural milk is poor in vitamin D, but milk in the U.S. is fortified with vitamin D.

However, even fortified milk contains only 100 I.U. per cup (8 oz or 240 ml).

Drink one to two cups a day. In this way, you get about 100-200 I.U. of vitamin D and other components of milk in a small to moderate amount. Milk is a good source of calcium. It's also a good source of protein and also contains some natural sugar and some fat.

Milk is a much better choice than soft drinks, which are loaded with sugar or other artificial sweeteners which can have a lot of side-effects. Diet drinks have no real nutritional value. Another disadvantage: soft drinks don't have any vitamin D.

People with lactose intolerance obviously should either drink Lactose free milk or avoid milk altogether.

YOGURT

Some yogurts have added vitamin D. Yogurt is also an excellent source of calcium as well as Lactobacillus, a friendly bacteria, which is very important for the health of your intestines.

CHEESE

Some cheeses contain a small amount of vitamin D. Cheeses are fattening and are also loaded with LDL (bad) cholesterol. I advise patients to limit cheeses to reduce weight and also to lower LDL cholesterol.

FISH

Oily fish such as salmon, mackerel and blue fish naturally contain reasonable amounts of vitamin D. The amount of vitamin D in fish remains unchanged if it is baked, but decreases about 50% if the fish is fried. Also, farm raised salmon has only about 25% of vitamin D as compared to wild salmon.

A word of caution about fish consumption!

Too much fish consumption can lead to mercury poisoning. Fish with high mercury content include shark, whale, swordfish, king mackerel, tilefish and tuna (both fresh and frozen tuna). However, canned tuna doesn't seem to be high in mercury because it consists of smaller, shorter-lived species. Fresh water fish which can be high in mercury include bass, pike, and muskellunge.

Therefore, I recommend caution when consuming fish. Moderation is the key. Avoid those fish that contain high levels of mercury. This is particularly true for pregnant women, lactating women, young children and women of child bearing age, as the developing brain of the fetus and newborn is very susceptible to the injurious effects of mercury. For this reason, the Food and Drug Administration recommends that pregnant women, breast feeding women and young children should avoid eating fish with high mercury content.

Other food items

Other foods that contain very small amounts of vitamin D include vegetables, meats and egg yolk. Most cereals in the U.S. are fortified with small amounts of vitamin D. Orange juice is also fortified with a small amount of vitamin D.

The following food items are supposed to contain the indicated amount of vitamin D:

- Salmon, cooked (3.5 ounces)   360 I.U.
- Mackerel, cooked (3.5 ounces)   345 I.U.
- Canned Tuna (3.0 ounces)   200 I.U.
- Sardines canned in oil, drained (1.75 ounces)   250 I.U.
- Raw shiitake mushroom (10 ounces)   76 I.U.
- Fortified milk, one cup (8 ounces or 240 ml)   100 I.U.
- Fortified Orange juice (8 ounces or 240 ml)   100 I.U.

- Fortified cereal, per serving   40-80 I.U.
- Egg, 1 whole (vitamin D is found in yolk)   20 I.U.
- Liver of beef, cooked   (3.5 ounces)   15 I.U.
- Swiss cheese (1 ounce)   12 I.U.

I.U. = International Units

A Word of Caution!

You can't simply rely on the stated quantities of vitamin D in a food item. For example, in one study, researchers found that vitamin D in milk was less than 80% of the stated amount (2). Also, vitamin D content of fish is highly variable.

3. Vitamin D supplements

From a practical perspective, you don't get enough vitamin D from sun exposure and food. Therefore, you need to take a vitamin D supplement. For most people, it becomes the major source of vitamin D.

The Starting Dose of Vitamin D Supplement ━━━━━

The starting dose of vitamin D supplement depends on how low your vitamin D level is. The aim is to build up your stores of vitamin D and then keep them well replenished. In most cases I start patients on Vitamin D3 (cholecalciferol). Only rarely do I use Vitamin D2 (ergocalciferol).

Here is an outline for how I choose the starting dose of vitamin D3 in my patients.

Vitamin D level (in ng/ml)	Starting dose of Vitamin D3 (in I.U.)
Less than 10	7000 I.U. a day
11 – 15	6000 I.U. a day
16 - 20	5000 I.U. a day
21- 25	3000 - 4000 I.U. a day
26 - 30	2000 - 3000 I.U. a day
31- 40	1000 - 2000 I.U. a day
More than 40	1000 I.U. a day

I.U. = International Units

Pay attention to the units on your vitamin D supplement!

In the U.S., the dose of vitamin D is available in I.U. However, in some parts of the world, vitamin D is available in microgram (mcg).

Here is the conversion factor:
40 I.U. = 1 mcg
For example: 400 I.U. = 10 mcg
                1000 I.U. = 25 mcg.
                50,000 I.U. = 1250 mcg or 1.25 mg

VITAMIN D2, 50,000 I.U.

When Vitamin D level is below 20, an alternative treatment is to take a high dose of vitamin D2. This is usually given as 50,000 I.U. per week for about 12 weeks. In the U.S., you need a physician's prescription for this dose of vitamin D2.

Recently, vitamin D3 also became available in a dose of 50,000 I.U.

The Maintenance Dose of Vitamin D Supplement ━━━━━━━

A common problem arises from traditional medical training which teaches that once your vitamin D stores are replenished, you go back to a daily maintenance dose of 400 I.U. a day. For example, if your vitamin D is very low (let's say less than 15 ng/ml), your physician will likely place you on a high dose of vitamin D2 such as 50,000 I.U. a week for 12 weeks and afterwards, put you back on 400 I.U. a day as a maintenance dose.

Most likely, in the following months, your physician won't check to see what happens to your vitamin D level on this miniscule dose. This kind of practice is based on the medical myth hammered into physicians that once you've replenished vitamin D stores, the problem is somehow cured.

Take a closer look at this myth. Vitamin D stays in your body stores for just a few weeks. Therefore, the "so called cure" of low vitamin D will only last a few weeks and then you'll be back to your usual state of a low level of vitamin D.

For this reason, I check vitamin D level in my patients every three months. What I've discovered is eye opening! In my clinical experience, the maintenance dose of vitamin D depends on the initial starting dose. For example, if a patient requires a high initial starting dose, that patient will need a high maintenance dose. Most people continue to require a high dose of vitamin D to maintain a good level. It makes perfect sense. Why?

It's the overall lifestyle of a person that determines the level of vitamin D. If a person is very low in vitamin D to begin with, it's due to his/her life-style, which in most cases doesn't change after a few weeks of vitamin D therapy. Therefore, it's important to continue a relatively high dose of vitamin D as a maintenance dose, especially in those individuals who are very low in vitamin D to start with.

Most of my patients require a daily dose of 2000-6000 I.U. of vitamin D3 to maintain a good level of vitamin D. Some need up to 8000-10,000 I.U. a day.

In general, obese people require a larger dose compared to thin people, as vitamin D is fat soluble and gets trapped in the fat.

CASE STUDY

Remember **Martin** from Chapter 10. At the time of diagnosis of colon cancer, his 25 (OH) vitamin D level was low as 20 ng/ml.

He was also obese. He needed to take 4000 I.U. of vitamin D3 per day to increase his 25 (OH) vitamin D level to 41 ng/ml. On his last visit, I increased his Vitamin D3 dose to 6000 I.U. per day to get his 25 (OH) vitamin D in the 50-100 ng/ml range.

CASE STUDY

When he came to see me, Damien was a 67 years old obese Caucasian male with vitamin D deficiency. His initial 25 (OH) vitamin D level was 23 ng/ml. Over the last 3 years, he has been on vitamin D3 ranging from 3000-4000 I.U. a day and his 25 (OH) vitamin D level has been in the mid 30's to mid 40's. Three months ago, I increased his dose to 6000 I.U. a day.

His most recent level of 25 (OH) vitamin D was 49 ng/ml.

Monitoring Vitamin D Level

I cannot overemphasize the need for close monitoring of your vitamin D level. An individual's response to a dose of vitamin D varies widely.

As I mentioned before, because vitamin D is fat soluble, it gets trapped in fat. That means there is less vitamin D available for the rest of the body. Therefore, obese people require a larger dose of vitamin D than lean individuals.

As vitamin D is fat soluble, it requires normal intestinal mechanisms to absorb fat. If a person has some problem with fat absorption, such as patients with chronic pancreatitis or pancreatic surgery or stomach surgery, then they may not absorb vitamin D adequately.

During summertime, the sun is stronger and many people spend time outdoors. Therefore, the required dose of vitamin D supplement may go down a bit. In wintertime, the dose of vitamin D may need to go up a bit. However, in a lot of individuals this seasonal variation is little as they mostly stay indoors and apply a good layer of sunscreen when they do go out.

The amount of vitamin D people get from their food also fluctuates considerably. In addition, some people take their vitamin D supplement regularly, while others take it sporadically.

Therefore, I check 25 (OH) vitamin D blood level every 3 months and adjust the dose of vitamin D accordingly. My aim is to achieve and maintain a level of 25 (OH) vitamin D in the range of 50-100 ng/ml (125-250 nmol/L).

I also check blood calcium to make sure that a person doesn't develop vitamin D toxicity. (See Chapter 24, Vitamin D Toxicity). I recommend monitoring vitamin D and blood calcium level every three months. The blood test for calcium is part of a chemistry panel, usually referred to as CHEM 12 (chemistry 12) or CMP (Comprehensive Metabolic Panel). It's a routine blood test for most people who have an ongoing health issue such as diabetes, hypertension, cholesterol disorder, arthritis, etc.

Special Situations ━━━━━━━━━━━━━━━

1. STEROIDS

Because steroids lower your vitamin D, I educate my patients to notify me if another doctor places them on a steroid. When someone takes a high dose steroid in an oral form such as Prednisone or in an injectable form such as Solumedrol, Depomedrol or Decadron, I increase the dose of vitamin D3 to 5000-8000 I.U. per day.

I check their 25 (OH) vitamin D level every 2 months and change the dose of vitamin D accordingly.

2. CHILDREN AND TEENAGERS

Because human milk doesn't contain any appreciable amounts of vitamin D, infants who are solely breastfed are at high risk for vitamin D deficiency. Therefore, the American Academy of Pediatrics recently raised their recommended daily dose of vitamin D to 400 I.U. in infants who are solely breastfed, beginning at the age of two months.

In most children a daily dose of vitamin D of 400-1000 I.U. seems appropriate. In addition, it makes sense to use sensible sun exposure, especially in infants and toddlers.

The teenage years are the time when most of your bone growth takes place. Therefore, teenagers need a good dose of vitamin D and calcium. In my opinion, they should be encouraged to spend time outdoors and have sensible sun exposure. In addition, they should also take vitamin D3 in a dose of 1000-2000 I.U. a day; 1000 I.U. for those who are lean and 2000 I.U. for those who are obese.

2. PREGNANT AND BREASTFEEDING WOMEN

These women are at higher risk for vitamin D deficiency. Low vitamin D in the mother leads to low vitamin D in the infant, with the terrible consequences mentioned in Chapter 19, Vitamin D Deficiency During Pregnancy and Breastfeeding. Therefore, for pregnant and breastfeeding women, I check vitamin D level at baseline and monitor it every two months. I treat their low vitamin D as described earlier in this chapter.

If blood levels aren't available, then these women should take a dose of at least 2000 I.U. of vitamin D3 a day.

4. MALABSORPTION SYNDROMES

Low vitamin D is extremely common among people with malabsorption syndromes such as Crohn's disease, Celiac sprue, chronic pancreatitis and intestinal, pancreatic or stomach surgeries. In these patients, early diagnosis and treatment of vitamin D deficiency is important or they end up developing another disease, secondary hyperparathyroidism. For details on secondary hyperparathyroidism, see Chapter 6.

In these patients, I check baseline vitamin D level. I find that it is almost always very low. I treat low vitamin D according to my strategy discussed earlier. These patients usually require a **large** dose of vitamin D to meet their vitamin D needs.

CASE STUDY

Andrea is a Caucasian female who developed cancer of the pancreas at the age of 59. Her surgeon removed 85% of her pancreas. Subsequently, she developed diabetes and came to see me. In addition to treating her diabetes, I also treated her vitamin D deficiency. She takes pancreatic enzyme supplements, but still requires large doses of vitamin D. Her most recent blood level of 25 (OH) vitamin D was 39 ng/ml while on a daily dose of 8000 I.U. of vitamin D3. Since then, I have increased her vitamin D3 dose to 10,000 I.U. a day

---

CASE STUDY

Remember **Jenny,** the 63 years old Caucasian female who underwent stomach bypass surgery? No one paid any attention to her vitamin D needs following her surgery. Three years later, when I got involved in her medical care, I found that she was severely low in vitamin D and had developed secondary hyperparathyroidism due to prolonged, severe vitamin D deficiency. To meet her vitamin D needs, she requires large doses of vitamin D. Currently, she is on 50,000 I.U. of vitamin D2 *every other day* and on this high dose, her most recent level of 25 (OH) vitamin D was only 29 ng/ml. Subsequently I have increased her dose to 50,000 I.U. of vitamin D *every day.*

REFERENCES:

1. Bischoff-Ferrari H et al. Current recommended vitamin D may not be optimal. *Am J Clin Nutr.* 2006;84:18-28.
2. Holick MF, Shao Q, Liu WW, et al. The vitamin D content of fortified milk and infant formula. *N Engl J Med.* 1992;326(18):1178-81.

CHAPTER 24

Vitamin D Toxicity

Every article written in newspapers and magazines about vitamin D always includes an overly scary caution about vitamin D toxicity. The reader gets the impression that it must be a common consequence of vitamin D supplementation. Some readers get so scared, they decide not to take vitamin D supplementation and end up with the health consequences of vitamin D deficiency. What a shame! It's obvious to me that the writers of these magazine and newspaper articles don't actually treat patients with low vitamin D and their knowledge about vitamin D toxicity is very limited and superficial.

What is Vitamin D toxicity?

Vitamin D toxicity is defined as "too much vitamin D, causing harm to the body."

What level of vitamin D causes damage to the body?

A blood level of 25 (OH) vitamin D consistently more than 200 ng/ml (500 nmol/L) is considered to be <u>potentially</u> toxic (1). Please note "potentially toxic." It means that there is a potential risk for vitamin D toxicity if your blood level is more than 200 ng/ml. However, it doesn't mean that you automatically suffer from vitamin D toxicity if you're above 200 ng/ml.

Indeed, in an animal model, blood concentration of vitamin D up to 400 ng/ml (1000 nmol/L) was not associated with any toxicity (2).

The experts in the field of vitamin D have chosen this cut off level of 200 ng/ml (500 nmol/L) arbitrarily in order to provide a safe limit. Please note that the normal range of 25 (OH) vitamin D is 30-100 ng/ml (75-250 nmol/L).

How Frequent is Vitamin D Toxicity?

Extremely rare.

I check vitamin D level in all of my patients and been doing so over the last ten years. In the last ten years, *I haven't seen a single case of serious vitamin D toxicity in my patients while they are on vitamin D3 or D2 supplementation!*

These patients are usually on a daily dose of 2000 I.U. to 6000 I.U. (50 mcg to 150 mcg) of vitamin D3, or a weekly dose of vitamin D2 of 50,000 I.U. (1.25 mg). None of these patients has had a level of 25 (OH) vitamin D above 100 ng/ml (250 nmol/L).

Rarely, I see a patient with a slight increase in calcium level above the normal limit. Simply reducing calcium intake brings the calcium back into the normal range in these patients. I don't consider this slight increase in the calcium level as a case of vitamin D toxicity.

My experience is in line with other experts in the field of vitamin D.

Risk of toxicity; Over the Counter Vitamin D3 versus Prescription Calcitriol (Rocaltrol).

Let me clarify another issue. When medical writers of newspaper and magazine articles talk of vitamin D toxicity, they make a blanket statement about vitamin D supplements which is a mistake. There are several different preparations of vitamin D supplements. These include Vitamin D3 (cholecalciferol), Vitamin D2 (ergocalciferol), Calcifediol and Calcitriol. Calcitriol is also known as the brand name Rocaltrol.

Calcitriol (Rocaltrol) is a synthetic form of vitamin D and is a drug rather than a supplement. Therefore, it requires a prescription from a physician. It is typically given to patients who have kidney failure and are on dialysis. Calcitriol (Rocaltrol) is also sometimes prescribed to patients whose parathyroid glands have been removed, often inadvertently by a surgeon during thyroid surgery.

Calcitriol (Rocaltrol) is much more potent than natural vitamin D3 or D2 and can sometimes result in vitamin D toxicity. Physicians who prescribe calcitriol (Rocaltrol) are typically aware (and definitely should be aware) of this possibility and monitor their patients for vitamin D toxicity.

Can You Develop Vitamin D Toxicity From Too Much Sun?

The answer is No. You can't develop vitamin D toxicity from too much sun exposure. The reason? Nature is smart. The skin forms as much vitamin D as the body needs. Beyond that, it degrades any excess vitamin D that is formed in the skin (3). Pretty smart!

How Do You Detect Vitamin D Toxicity?

Vitamin D helps in the absorption of calcium from the intestines. Toxic levels of Vitamin D can cause an increase in blood level of calcium. Thus, vitamin D toxicity manifests itself as a high level of calcium in the blood.

The simplest and the most scientific way to find vitamin D toxicity is to check your calcium and vitamin D level in the blood. Everyone should have his/her vitamin D level and calcium checked every three months. If your 25(OH) Vitamin D level is higher than 100 ng/ml (250 nmol/L) or your blood calcium gets elevated, then you should reduce your dose of vitamin D. However, please note that you are still way below the potentially toxic level of 200 ng/ml (500 nmol/L).

Symptoms of Vitamin D Toxicity

Symptoms of vitamin D toxicity are due to increase in the blood level of calcium.

Mild increase in blood calcium level
Usually doesn't cause any symptoms.

Moderate increase in blood calcium
Usually causes non-specific symptoms of nausea, vomiting, constipation, poor appetite, weight loss and weakness. Remember these symptoms can be caused by a variety of other medical conditions as well.

Severe increase in blood calcium level
Causes neurologic symptoms such as somnolence, confusion, even coma and heart rhythm abnormalities which can be fatal if not treated promptly.

Treatment for Vitamin D Toxicity

Rarely, I see a patient whose blood calcium goes slightly above the upper limit of normal while on vitamin D supplementation. I lower their calcium intake and repeat a blood test for calcium in a month. In my experience, the reduction in calcium intake brings down calcium into the normal range.

Very rarely, blood calcium remains slightly elevated. I then check parathyroid hormone level. If it is in the normal range, then I further discuss diet with the patient and try to lower calcium intake. Even in these very rare patients, blood calcium normalizes by lowering their calcium intake.

I also keep in mind other causes for elevated blood calcium level such as primary hyperparathyroidism and cancer. I order diagnostic testing in this regard on a case by case basis.

If blood calcium is elevated and parathyroid hormone (PTH, intact) is also elevated and both of these values do not normalize with vitamin D supplementation, then that patient is most likely suffering from primary hyperparathyroidism.

If parathyroid hormone (PTH, intact) level is normal and the patient continues to have an elevated calcium level, I investigate the possibility of other causes of high calcium such as cancer.

Rarely, high blood calcium may occur due to vitamin D toxicity which can happen if very high doses of vitamin D are used (such as 50,000 I.U. per day) for a long period, although I have not seen it in my practice.

In my experience, the usual doses of vitamin D3 ranging from 2000 I.U. to 6000 I.U. per day, do not cause a high blood calcium level.

Remember, there are many causes of an increase in blood calcium level other than vitamin D toxicity. Two such common causes of high blood calcium are: Primary hyperparathyroidism and cancer. If you have high blood calcium, your physician should thoroughly look into various causes of high blood calcium.

It's important to notify your physician about all the dietary supplements, including vitamin D, which you take. Most physicians don't specifically ask about dietary supplements and often patients don't think to provide this information either. For best medical care, your physician should know all the medicines as well as all the dietary supplements that you take.

If your physician determines that a mild increase in your blood calcium level is due to excessive doses of "over the counter" vitamin D supplementation, as evidenced by a high blood level of 25(OH) vitamin D, in consultation with your physician, you should decrease the dose of your calcium intake and vitamin D. In most cases, simply reducing the calcium intake will bring calcium back into the normal range. If your physician advises you to reduce the dose of vitamin D, you should do so.

Recheck your calcium level in a month or so to make sure that your blood calcium is back to normal. Recheck your vitamin D and calcium in about 3 months to make sure that these levels are good and you haven't swung in the other direction.

If your blood calcium is high due to "prescription vitamin D", such as **calcitriol**, the treatment will depend upon the degree of high blood calcium and your symptoms. Your physician will manage it accordingly. If your calcium level is moderate to severely high, your physician will likely admit you to the hospital for proper treatment of vitamin D toxicity.

REFERENCES:

1. Jones G. The pharmacokinetics of vitamin D. *Am J Clin Nutr.* In press.
2. Shepard RM, DeLuca HF. Plasma concentrations of vitamin D3 and its metabolites in the rat as influenced by vitamin D3 or 245-hydoxyvitamin D3 intakes. *Arch Biochem Biophys* 1980;202:43-53.
3. Holick MF. Vitamin D deficiency. *N Engl J Med* 2007;357:266-81.

In Summary

In recent years, we've discovered that vitamin D is not only important for the health of the bones, but plays a crucial role in the health of almost every organ system in the body. Vitamin D may play an important role for the *prevention as well as treatment* of chronic fatigue, muscle aches and pains, cancer, diabetes, heart disease, high blood pressure, osteoporosis, immune disorders, kidney failure, dental problems, skin disorders and depression. Unfortunately, most people are not benefitting from these miraculous effects of vitamin D. Why? Because most people are low in vitamin D!

We are facing an epidemic of vitamin D deficiency. The main reasons for this epidemic are our modern life-style, misconceptions about vitamin D and the outdated daily recommended dose of vitamin D contained in daily vitamins and calcium formulas.

Vitamin D deficiency can be easily diagnosed with a simple blood test, 25 (OH) vitamin D. Most physicians make the mistake of ordering 1,25 $(OH)_2$ vitamin D instead, which is the *wrong test* to diagnose vitamin D deficiency. Why is it the wrong test? Because it's often normal and may even be high in people who are actually suffering from vitamin D deficiency.

The only good natural source of vitamin D is the sun. How much vitamin D your skin can synthesize from sun exposure depends upon several factors such as latitude, season, time of the day, color of the skin, age, sun screen lotions, air pollution and shade. You need a significant amount of sun exposure on naked skin to get enough vitamin D from the sun. This degree of sun exposure poses a significant risk of skin cancer.

Food items contain very small amounts of vitamin D.

The best way to get an optimal level of vitamin D is sensible sun exposure and a vitamin D supplement. Most physicians don't know the dosage amount of vitamin D supplement to recommend.

Based upon my extensive clinical experience, I recommend vitamin D3 in a daily dose of 2000-6000 I.U. (50-150 microgram) for most of my patients. I aim for an optimal blood level of 25 (OH) vitamin D in the range of 50-100 ng/ml (125-250 nmol/L). I check 25 (OH) vitamin D and calcium blood level in my patients every three months to ensure they achieve an optimal level of vitamin D and maintain it. By employing this strategy, I achieve a good level of vitamin D while preventing vitamin D toxicity. In my extensive experience, I have *not* encountered any vitamin D toxicity in my patients on vitamin D 3 or vitamin D2 supplements.

By employing my unique, scientific approach to diagnose and treat vitamin D deficiency, I am seeing great health benefits in my patients. Nothing can be more rewarding! You too, can benefit from this strategy, but you should do so with the blessing of your own health care provider. Good luck in taking charge of your vitamin D needs!

Sarfraz Zaidi, MD
www.DoctorZaidi.com

ACKNOWLEDGEMENTS

I gratefully acknowledge Georgie Huntington Zaidi, my editor, who did an extraordinary job of transforming this complex medical book into an easy read. On a personal note, I am so grateful to Georgie for being my wonderful wife.

I am also grateful to our lovely daughter, Zareena, for listening to our advice about vitamin D and other health as well as life issues.

I also sincerely appreciate Dolly Zaidi for her in-depth proof reading.

I am deeply grateful to my wonderful patients who graciously granted me permission to include their case studies without which, the book would have been *colorless*.

I also sincerely acknowledge the brilliant scientific work of many researchers devoted to the field of vitamin D.

Sarfraz Zaidi, M.D.
www.DoctorZaidi.com

Conversion Table

Reference values to convert various systems in the world regarding the blood level and daily dose of vitamin D.

Blood level of 25 (OH) Vitamin D
1 ng /ml = 2.5 nmol/L
30 ng/ml = 75 nmol/L
100 ng/ml = 250 nmol/L

*ng = nanogram ml = milliliter nmol = nanomole L = liter

Vitamin D Dose
40 I.U. = 1 mcg
400 I.U. = 10 mcg
1000 I.U. = 25 mcg
50,000 I.U. = 1250 mcg or 1.25 mg

*I.U. = International Unit   mcg = microgram   mg = milligram

CPSIA information can be obtained at www.ICGtesting.com
Printed in the USA
LVOW100559201011

251324LV00002B/20/P